Workbook with Lab Exercises to Accompany
Principles of Radiographic Imaging: An Art and a Science

2nd edition

William F. Finney, III, M.A., R.T.(R)
Acting Director and Assistant Professor
School of Allied Medical Professions
The Ohio State University
Columbus, Ohio

Richard R. Carlton, M.S., R.T.(R)(CV), FAERS
Chairman of Diagnostic Medical Imaging
City College of San Francisco
San Francisco, California

Arlene M. Adler, M.Ed., R.T.(R), FAERS
Director, Radiologic Sciences
Indiana University Northwest
Gary, Indiana

Correlated to **Principles of Radiographic Imaging: An Art and a Science,** 2nd edition
by Richard R. Carlton and Arlene M. Adler

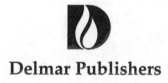

Delmar Publishers

I(T)P An International Thomson Publishing Company

Albany • Bonn • Boston • Cincinnati • Detroit • London • Madrid • Melbourne
Mexico City • New York • Pacific Grove • Paris • San Francisco • Singapore • Tokyo
Toronto • Washington

Notice to the Reader

Copyright © 1996
By Delmar Publishers
A division of International Thomson Publishing Inc.

The ITP logo is a trademark under license

Printed in the United States of America

Delmar Publishers' Online Services
To access Delmar on the World Wide Web, point your browser to: http://www.delmar.com/delmar.html
To access through Gopher: gopher://gopher.delmar.com
(Delmar Online is part of "thomson.com", an Internet site with information on more than 30 publishers of the International Thomson Publishing organization.)
For information on our products and services: email info@delmar.com or call 800-347-7707

For more information, contact:

Delmar Publishers
3 Columbia Circle, Box 15015
Albany, New York 12212-5015

International Thomson Publishing Europe
Berkshire House 168-173
High Holborn
London WC1V7AA
England

Thomas Nelson Australia
102 Dodds Street
South Melbourne, 3205
Victoria, Australia

Nelson Canada
1120 Birchmount Road
Scarborough, Ontario
Canada M1K 5G4

International Thomson Editores
Campos Eliseos 385, Piso 7
Col Polanco
11560 Mexico D F Mexico

International Thomson Publishing GmbH
Königswinterer Strasse 418
53227 Bonn
Germany

International Thomson Publishing Asia
221 Henderson Road
#05–10 Henderson Building
Singapore 0315

International Thomson Publishing – Japan
Hirakawacho Kyowa Building, 3F
2–2–1 Hirakawacho
Chiyoda-ku, Tokyo 102
Japan

3 4 5 6 7 8 9 10 XXX 02 01 00 99 98 97

Library of Congress Card Number: 95–48883

ISBN: 0–8273–6866–6

Dedicated to

Mary Carol, Todd, and Zane Finney

Meredith and Katie Adler

Michelle, Kristöfer, Ærik, Edward, and Michael Carlton

TABLE OF CONTENTS

UNIT I   CREATING THE BEAM

UNIT II   PROTECTING PATIENTS AND PERSONNEL

UNIT III   CREATING THE IMAGE

UNIT IV   ANALYZING THE IMAGE

UNIT VI   SPECIAL IMAGING SYSTEMS

PREFACE

This workbook has been designed to correlate with the textbook **Principles of Radiographic Imaging: An Art and A Science,** 2nd edition. Our intent has been to design a series of activities, both laboratories and worksheets, to provide higher level synthesis and analysis activities for each chapter in the textbook. There are 93 exercises, of which 72 are laboratories and 21 are worksheets. There is at least one exercise for each text chapter, with multiple activities for chapters that require exercises to assist students in understanding the more difficult concepts.

This workbook represents a correlated series of exercises to help strengthen didactic instruction. There are sufficient activities to support a regularly scheduled laboratory for courses in physics, principles of exposure, and imaging. An equipment chart is provided to assist faculty in preparing for each laboratory and for ordering supplies and equipment prior to each course.

Students are expected to be able to operate radiographic equipment, a film processor, densitometer, sensitometer, oscilloscope, and dosimeter for various exercises. No worksheets or laboratories are provided to teach students the operation of this equipment as we found wide differences in manufacturers' operating instructions. We suggest that students be shown how to operate each new piece of equipment at the start of the laboratory where it must be used. Alternatively, faculty may produce laboratory exercises for this purpose by duplicating the relevant portions of the manufacturer's operating manual.

Bill is the primary author of this workbook although Rick and Arlene made numerous contributions. Many of the exercises were based on laboratories that have been in use for many years at The Ohio State University, Lima Technical College, and Indiana University Northwest. Bill also designed a number of exercises specifically for the chapters in the textbook. All of the activities were tested in our labs and found to be sound in concept. Additional testing was done by Barry Burns at the University of North Carolina. Each activity has a set of instructions with reasonable equipment requirements and preparation time.

We acknowledge responsibility for all errors in content. It is the responsibility of faculty to properly prepare students for laboratory coursework and therefore we assume no responsibility for damage to equipment or persons as a result of students performing these exercises. In addition, information in this workbook should only be used in clinical practice subservient to prevailing procedures and under the direction of appropriate supervisory personnel.

ACKNOWLEDGMENTS

We owe special thanks to our editor Marjorie Bruce at Delmar, our students, especially those at Lima Technical College, The Ohio State University, and Indiana University Northwest who patiently worked through the revisions of these laboratories under the direction of Andy Shappell and Wil Reddinger (LTC), Barb Hanna, Chris Hornback, and Sue Woods (IUN). Their special delight in finding our errors is greatly appreciated.

William Finney, Columbus, Ohio
Richard Carlton, Lima, Ohio
Arlene Adler, Gary, Indiana
September, 1995

EXPOSURE TECHNIQUE FACTORS

The use of these laboratories requires fine adjustment of exposure technical factors for each exercise. Most of the experiments that use radiographic film are based on the use of a 400 relative speed film/screen combination. Because of the complex variations in diagnostic imaging systems, it is impossible to suggest exposure factors that will produce ideal results in all situations. Faculty members may wish to produce the films for each experiment in order to obtain exact technical factors prior to assigning the laboratories to students. Alternately, if students are working individually or in small groups, the entire group may learn valuable lessons by assisting in adjusting our suggested factors until an ideal density has been achieved for each activity. In all cases, the **image density should be adjusted by mAs changes only** (unless otherwise stated in the laboratory instructions). **Kilovoltage levels have been chosen for specific effects in many experiments and should not be changed unless absolutely necessary due to equipment limitations.**

LABORATORY EQUIPMENT AND MATERIALS

The majority of laboratory activities contained in this manual require specific items that are common to a radiography environment. In order to facilitate the instructor and student in preparing for the laboratory activities, the following equipment/materials matrix lists the basic equipment and material requirements for each laboratory experiment. For a more complete description of the recommended items, the reader should refer to the specific laboratory experiment. Laboratories listed with a # sign indicate items with alternative choices or options for completion of the experiment. Those listed with a * sign indicate that the items have to be prepared or constructed prior to the experiment. Refer to the specific experiment for detailed instructions. Keep in mind that the equipment/materials recommendations have been made based on field trials and are not etched in stone, so feel free to substitute the equipment and/or material items if deemed necessary. Remember that ingenuity is the mother of all experiments.

3–1	3–2	4–1	4–2
Electroscope	1.5 V battery	#9 V battery (dry cell)	#Ammeter
Static rods	or DC power source	Bar magnets	Bar magnets
Silk patches	Ammeter/Voltmeter	Cardboard	Galvanometer or ammeter
Wool patches	Copper wire	Compass	*Wire helix coils
	Resistors (Five 5 watt)	Galvanometer or	Copper wire with alligator
		ammeter	clips
		Iron filings	
		Wire	

5–2	6–1	8–1	9–1
Cable/BNC connectors	X-ray tube parts	Dosimeter	Dosimeter
Radiographic unit		Phantom body part	Gonad shields
Storage oscilloscope		Radiographic unit	Phantom body part
X-ray output detector		Ring stand	Radiographic unit
			Ring stand

10–1	10–2	11–2	13–1
0.25, 0.5, 1.0, 2.0 mm	Radiographic unit	Dosimeter	Digital dosimeter
Al filters	4 1 mm Al attenuators	Radiographic unit	Radiographic unit
Radiographic unit	Dosimeter		Technique chart
Dosimeter			

14–1	15–1	16–1	17–1
Cassette/film	Cassette/film	Cassette/film	Teaching radiographs
Dosimeter	Film processor	Cassette holder	
Film processor	Phantom body part	Dosimeter	
Phantom body part	Plastic gallon jugs	Film processor	
Radiographic unit	Radiographic unit	Phantom body part	
		Radiographic unit	
		Wire mesh tool	

18–1

Aluminum step wedge
Cassette/film
Densitometer
Film processor
Phantom body part
8:1 and 12:1 grids
Radiographic unit

18–2

Cassette/film
Film processor
Phantom body part
12:1 grid
Radiographic unit

18–3

Cassette/film
Densitometer
Film processor
Phantom body part
Radiographic unit

19–2

Densitometer
Duplication film
Duplication unit
Film processor
Radiograph, good quality
Radiograph, overexposed

19–3

Densitometer
Film processor
Radiographs, angiography
  study
Subtraction mask film
Subtraction print film
Subtraction unit

20–1

Densitometer
Film processor
Radiographic film
Sensitometer
Thermometer

20–2

Film processor

21–1

Densitometer
Film processor
Graph paper
Radiographic film
Sensitometer

22–1

Aluminum step wedge
Densitometer
Film processor
Radiographic unit
Various intensifying
  screens in cassette

22–2

Cassette/film
Empty film box
Film processor
Hand lotion
Lighter

23–1

Aluminum step wedge
Cassettes/films (variety)
Densitometer
Dosimeter
Film processor
Phantom body part
Radiographic unit
Resolution test tool

24–1

Radiographic unit
Phantom body part
Cassette

25–1

Aluminum step wedge
Cassette/film
Densitometer
Film processor
Phantom body part
Radiographic unit

25–2

Aluminum step wedge
Cassette/film
Densitometer
Film processor
Phantom body part
Radiographic unit

25–3

Cassette/film
Densitometer
Film processor
Phantom body part

25–4

Aluminum step wedge
Cassette/film
Densitometer
Film processor
Phantom body part
Radiographic unit

25–5

Aluminum step wedge
Densitometer
Film processor
Phantom body part
Radiographic unit
Various speed cassettes
  with film

25–6

1" Super ball
35 mm film canister
Barium solution
3"–4" container
Cassette/film
Film processor
Ice cubes
Radiographic unit
Note: These films are also
used for Laboratory 26–3

26–1

Aluminum step wedge
Cassette/film
Densitometer
Film processor
Phantom body part
Radiographic unit

26–2

Aluminum step wedge
Densitometer
Film processor
Radiographic unit
Various speed cassettes
  with film

26–3

Use films or supplies
from 25–6

26–4

Cassette/film
Film processor
Phantom body part
Radiographic unit

26–5

Aluminum step wedge
Cassette/film
Densitometer
Film processor
Phantom body part
Radiographic grids
Radiographic unit

27–1

Cassette/film
Dry bones
Film processor
Radiographic unit
Resolution pattern
Sponges
Lead masks

27–2

Cassette/film
Dry bones
Film processor
Radiographic unit
Resolution pattern
Sponges

27–3

Film processor
Phantom body part
Radiographic unit
Resolution pattern
Sponge
Various speed cassettes
with film

27–4

Non-screen film
holder/film
Film processor
Phantom body part
Radiographic unit
String

28–1

Cassette/film
Small dry bone (vertebrae
preferred)
Film processor
Metric ruler
Radiographic unit

28–2

Cassette/film
Dry bones
Film processor
Metric ruler
Radiographic unit

29–1

Repeated radiographs

30–1

Densitometer
Film processor
Sensitometer
Radiographic film
Thermometer

30–2

Non-screen film
holder/film
Film processor
Metric ruler
Radiographic unit
Star test pattern

30–3

Beam perpendicularity
test tool
Cassette/film
#Collimator test tool
Film processor
Nine pennies
Radiographic unit
with PBL
Scrap film
Paper clips

30–7

Digital dosimeter
Radiographic unit

30–4

Cassette/film
Coin
Film processor
Metric ruler
Radiographic unit
Ring stand
Scrap film
Bubble level
Angulator
Quarter

30–8

Adhesive tape
Cassettes, empty
Cassette/film
Film processor
Gauze pads
Radiographic unit
Screen cleaner
Wire mesh test tool

30–5

#Densitometer
Digital kVp meter
Film processor
#kVp test cassette (with
current calibration chart)
Radiographic unit

30–9

Light meter
View boxes
*View box test template

30–6

Cassette/film
Film processor
#Manual spin top
Protractor
Radiographic unit
Synchronous spin top

30–10

Repeated radiographs

WORKSHEET 1–1   **BASIC MATHEMATICS REVIEW**

PURPOSE

Drill and practice in solving basic mathematical problems.

ACTIVITIES

Carry out the math operations indicated and solve the following problems:

PROBLEMS FOR FRACTIONS

1. 1/9 + 4/9 =

2. 4/9 - 2/9 =

3. 2/5 ÷ 3/4 =

4. 3/4 · 1/5 =

5. 2/3 ÷ 5/7 =

PROBLEMS FOR DECIMALS

1. (34.21) · (1.1) =

2. 714.58 + 214.785 =

3. 725 ÷ 0.25 =

4. Change 85% to a decimal.

5. Change .081 to a percent.

PROBLEMS FOR COMPUTATION WITH VALUES (NUMBERS)

1. Round each of the following to the number of significant digits indicated.

    a. 328.14 (4)

    b. 1.25   (2)

    c. 2709   (3)

2. Multiply or divide the following numbers, leaving the result with the correct number of significant digits if each number is assumed to be approximate.

    a. (2.32)(1.2)

    b. (43.81) ÷ (2.23)

3. Multiply or divide the following numbers, leaving the result with the correct number of significant digits if each number is assumed to be approximate.

    a. (38.42)(3.82)

    b. (4.32) ÷ (1.5)

4. Add or subtract the following numbers, leaving the result with the correct number of significant digits if each number is assumed to be approximate.

    a. 21.3 + 21.39

    b. 48.61 + 61

5. How many significant digits are in each of the following?

   a. 7.04

   b. 180

   c. 180.0

   d. 9300

   e. 8104.6

PROBLEMS FOR SCIENTIFIC NOTATION

1. Change the following numbers to scientific notation.

   a. 784.2

   b. .00431

   c. 78,210,000

   d. .0000067

   e. 7.4

2. Change the following numbers to ordinary notation.

   a. 2.84×10^5

   b. 2.84×10^{-5}

   c. 6.18×10^0

   d. 6.18×10^{-2}

   e. 6.18×10^1

PROBLEMS FOR SIGNED NUMBERS

1. $(-6) - (-9) + (-6) =$

2. $(-8)(-2)(-3) =$

3. $(15) \div (-13) =$

4. $-6 - 8 - 2 + 3 =$

5. $(-2)(-1)(-1)(-1) =$

PROBLEMS FOR ORDER OF OPERATION

1. Evaluate each of the following:

   a. $17 - 8.2 + 4 \cdot 5 - 2.6^2$

   b. $(3+1)^2 - 4(8+2) - 5 \cdot (-1)$

   c. $6(2^2 - 4 \cdot 1) - 4^2$

   d. $-2(3 + 4 \cdot 5)$

   e. $(-8)^2 + 3 \cdot 5^2$

2. Evaluate each of the following:

   a. $7 + 4 \cdot 5$

   b. $6 \cdot 7 - 4 \cdot (-6)$

c. $2 \cdot 7^2$

d. $(-4)^2$

e. -4^2

f. $6(7+3) + 4 \cdot 8 - 7^2$

PROBLEMS FOR ALGEBRAIC EXPRESSIONS

1. Simplify the following algebraic expressions.

    a. $2(3x + 4y) + (x-y)$

    b. $2(x-4y) - 6(x+2y)$

    c. $6[2x-4(x-y)]$

    d. $-3[2(x+5y) - 6(2x +3y)]$

2. Simplify the following algebraic expressions.

    a. $2(3x + 4y) + (x-y)$

    b. $3(x-2y) - 6(x+y)$

    c. $4[3x-2(2x-3y)]$

    d. $8[-2(2x+3) + 4(x-y)]$

PROBLEMS FOR EXPONENTS

1. Simplify each of the following expressions leaving the answer with only positive exponents.

    a. $a^4 \cdot a^5 \cdot a^3$

    b. $\dfrac{b^8 \cdot b^4}{b^5}$

    c. $(a^2)^3 (b^{-2})^{-5}$

    d. $\dfrac{a^4 b^2 a^8 b^6}{a^5 b^3 a^{10} b^2}$

2. Simplify each of the following expressions leaving the answer with only positive exponents.

    a. $a^2 \cdot a^4 \cdot a^8$

    b. $\dfrac{b^6 b^2}{b^5}$

    c. $a^2 \cdot b^5 \cdot a^5 \cdot b^2$

    d. $\dfrac{a^8 b^{10}}{a^{11} b^4}$

PROBLEMS FOR EVALUATING ALGEBRAIC EXPRESSIONS

1. Evaluate each of the following expressions for $a = 5$, $b = 3$, and $c = -2$.

    a. $a + b \cdot c$

    b. $a + b - c$

    c. $2c + 3b^2 + 2(a-c)$

2. Evaluate each of the following expressions for $a = 2$, $b = -4$, and $c = 6$.

    a. $2a + 3b - 4c$

b. $b^2 - 2c^2 + a^2$

c. $5(a+2b-c) + 4 \cdot b$

PROBLEMS FOR EQUATIONS

1.   Solve for x: $\dfrac{x}{6} = 3$

2.   Solve for y: $2y + 3 = 9$

3.   Solve for b: $2(b + 6) = b + 12$

4.   Solve for x: $\dfrac{18}{11} \times \dfrac{3}{x}$

5.   Solve for a: $3(a + 4) = 15$

WORKSHEET 1-2   UNITS OF MEASUREMENT

PURPOSE

Drill and practice in solving units of measurement and dimensional analysis problems.

ACTIVITIES

Carry out the math operations indicated and solve the following problems:

PROBLEMS FOR DIMENSIONAL ANALYSIS

1. Convert 15 inches to yards.

2. Convert 1,500 seconds to hours.

3. Convert 1.8 hours to seconds.

4. Convert 18.9 feet to inches.

5. Convert 60 miles/hour to feet/second.

6. Convert 44 feet/second to miles/hour.

7. Convert 10 feet^2 to inches^2.

8. Convert 10 meters^2 to centimeters^2.

9. Convert 14 inches^3 to feet^3.

10. Convert 15 yards^3 to feet^3.

11. Convert 15.8 g/cm^3 to kg/m^3.

12. Convert 6.8 gallons to pints.

Identify the SI unit of measurement and symbol for the following quantities:

Quantity	UNIT	SYMBOL
13. Length	_____	_____
14. Mass	_____	_____
15. Time	_____	_____
16. Exposure	_____	_____
17. Absorbed Dose	_____	_____
18. Dose Equivalent	_____	_____

19. Convert 500 milliroentgens to coulombs/kilogram.

20. Convert 20 millirem to sieverts.

21. Convert 50 rads to grays.

22. Convert 6.45×10^{-4} coulombs/kilogram to Roentgens.

23. Convert 0.084 sievert to rems.

24. Convert 0.35 gray to rads.

PURPOSE

Describe the basic theory of atomic structure.

ACTIVITIES

1. How do atoms differ from molecules? elements from compounds?

2. List the three basic subatomic particles along with their corresponding mass number and charge.

3. What is the difference between a neutral atom and an ion?

4. How is the identity of an element determined?

5. What is the difference between atomic number, mass number, and atomic weight?

6. Draw a diagram of an aluminum atom.

7. How many valence electrons does aluminum have?

8. Name two elements that have a single valence electron.

9.   Identify the number of orbital shells for each of the following atoms:

   a. helium

   b. lead

   c. barium

   d. calcium

   e. oxygen

10.   What is the maximum number of electrons that can occupy the K shell? L shell? M shell? N shell? O shell? P shell? Q shell?

11.   Explain the octet rule.

12.   What do all of the elements in Group 1 of the periodic table have in common?

13.   What is the difference between an ionic and a covalent bond?

14.   Draw a diagram of a water molecule.

LABORATORY 3-1   **LAWS OF ELECTROSTATICS AND ELECTRODYNAMICS**

PURPOSE

Interpret the results of various electrostatic interactions.

MATERIALS

1.   Electroscope
2.   Static conducting rods or plastic strips
3.   Small pieces of wool and silk

PROCEDURES

1.   Always ground the electroscope by gently touching the knob with the palm of your hand prior to performing any experiment. If your electroscope has thin metal leaves, never touch them.

2.   Use a piece of cloth to rub your conducting strip, then touch the knob of the electroscope. Record your observations. Repeat for each type of cloth available.

3.   Use a piece of cloth to rub your conducting strip, then bring the conducting strip close to, but do not allow it to touch the knob of the electroscope. Record your observations. Repeat for each type of cloth available.

RESULTS

1.   Record the reaction that was observed in the electroscope for each type of cloth when the conducting rod or strip touched the knob.

2.   Record the reaction that was observed in the electroscope for each type of cloth when the conducting rod or strip came near, but did not touch, the knob.

ANALYSIS

Use − signs to indicate the presence of electrons. Do not use any + signs.

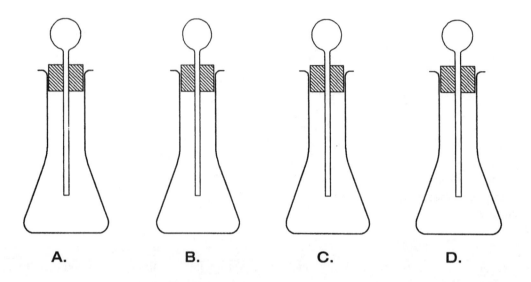

A.   B.   C.   D.

1. Use Figure A to indicate the distribution of electrons and the position of the leaves while a charged conducting rod was in contact with the knob.

2. Use Figure B to indicate the distribution of electrons and the position of the leaves after a charged rod was removed from contact with the knob.

3. Use Figure C to indicate the distribution of electrons and the position of the leaves while a charged rod was near, but not touching, the knob.

4. Use Figure D to indicate the distribution of electrons and the position of the leaves after a charged rod was removed from proximity with the knob.

5. Were there any differences in the effect seen with the various cloths? Why?

6. Which law of electrostatics was demonstrated in Figure A?

7. What is the term for the effect seen in Figure B?

8. What effect would be seen if the electroscope was subjected to an intense dose of ionizing radiation.

LABORATORY 3-2 _____ **OHM'S LAW AND RESISTANCE**

PURPOSE

Demonstrate the relationships involved in Ohm's Law.

MATERIALS

1. DC variable power source (five 1.5 volt C or D size batteries can be substituted)
2. Five 10 Ω, 5 watt resistors
3. Meters capable of measuring 0–10 V and 0–1,000 mA (0–1 A)
4. Connecting wires

PROCEDURES

THE EFFECT OF EMF ON CURRENT FLOW

1. Connect two 10 Ω resistors in series and hook the combination in series with an ammeter and the power source. Use a voltmeter across the power source to set it at 1.5 V. Record the applied voltage and the current flow as measured by the ammeter (in the range of 75 mA).

2. Repeat step 1 four more times after increasing the voltage in increments of 1.5 volts up to a total of 7.5 volts while leaving the resistance the same.

THE EFFECT OF RESISTANCE ON CURRENT FLOW

1. Use a voltmeter connected across the power source to adjust it to 6 V. Connect one 10 Ω resistor in series with the ammeter and hook the combination in series with the power source. Record the current measured by the ammeter (in the range of 600 mA).

2. Repeat step 1 for resistance values of 20, 30, 40, and 50 Ω by connecting in turn two, three, four, and five of the 10 Ω resistors in series.

RESULTS

THE EFFECT OF VOLTAGE ON CURRENT FLOW

1. Plot the following graph of current (I) against applied voltage (V) using the data obtained from steps 1 and 2. (Mark the vertical axis with mA values that will permit all your data to be graphed.)

GRAPH 1

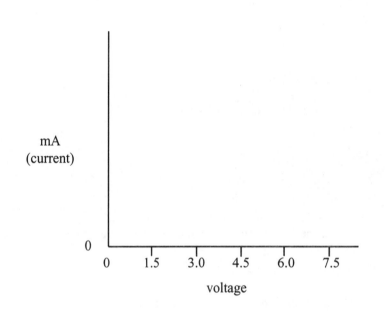

THE EFFECT OF RESISTANCE ON CURRENT FLOW

1. Plot the following graph of current (I) against resistance (R) voltage using the data obtained from steps 1 and 2. (Mark the vertical axis with mA values that will permit all your data to be graphed.)

GRAPH 2

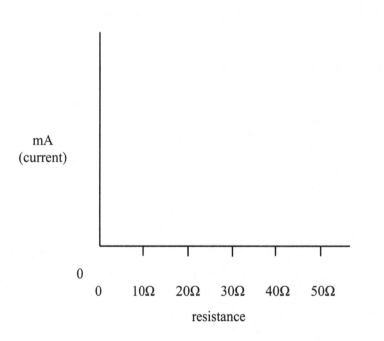

ANALYSIS

OHM'S LAW

Use Ohm's Law to fill in the missing quantities in the chart.

	amps	volts	ohms
1.	100	_____	4
2.	56	_____	312
3.	_____	110	60
4.	_____	2,110	11.5
5.	50	110	_____
6.	0.8	39	_____

EFFECT OF SERIES AND PARALLEL CIRCUITS ON RESISTANCE, CURRENT, AND EMF

7. What is the total resistance of a circuit if it contains resistances of 3 Ω, 2 Ω, and 10 Ω in series? in parallel?

8. What is the total resistance of a circuit if it contains resistances of 110 Ω, 26.2 Ω, and 14 Ω in series? in parallel?

9. If a circuit has resistances of 10 Ω, 12 Ω, and 2.4 Ω and an emf of 140 volts, what is the current if the circuit has the resistances in series? in parallel?

10. If a circuit has resistances of 10 Ω, 4.2 Ω, and 3 Ω and a current of 56 amps, what is the emf if the circuit has the resistances in series? in parallel?

13

THE EFFECT OF VOLTAGE ON CURRENT FLOW

11. Based on the results of the experiment as shown on graph 1, when the resistance was relatively constant, what effect did voltage have on amperage? Is this finding consistent with Ohm's Law?

THE EFFECT OF RESISTANCE ON CURRENT FLOW

12. Based on the results of the experiment as shown on graph 2, when the voltage was relatively constant, what effect did resistance have on amperage? Is this finding consistent with Ohm's Law?

LABORATORY 4-1   LAWS OF MAGNETISM AND MAGNETIC INDUCTION

PURPOSE

Demonstrate basic laws of magnetism, map static and dynamic field flux lines, and illustrate the basic principle of magnetic induction.

MATERIALS

1. Two bar magnets
2. Three pieces of stiff paper, cardboard, or Plexiglas (approximately 8" x 10")
3. Iron filings
4. 3' length of wire
5. Low voltage power supply or dry cell (about 9 V)
6. Compass
7. Galvanometer (or ammeter)

PROCEDURES

LAWS OF MAGNETISM

1. Place the two bar magnets end to end with both S poles about 3" apart. Hold both magnets tightly and bring the two ends together.

2. Repeat step 1 with a N and S pole together.

3. Repeat step 2 but hold the magnets away from each other at a distance of 2", 1", 1/2" while feeling the force of the magnetic field at each distance. Record the distances in order of magnetic field strength.

MAPPING A STATIC FIELD

1. Level paper with spacers to permit bar magnet to be positioned underneath.

2. Sprinkle iron filings on paper over magnet.

MAPPING A DYNAMIC FIELD

3. Run a wire vertically through a hole in the center of the paper (as shown in the figure). Connect the ends of a low voltage battery (9 volt dry cell suggested).

4. Draw arrows on the paper to map the direction of a compass needle (as shown in textbook Fig. 4-6). Place the compass on the surface of the paper and draw an arrow representing the direction of the compass needle. Slowly move the compass in a circle around the wire, adding arrows as the compass needle changes direction.

5. Reverse the connections of the wire at the battery and repeat step 4.

MAGNETIC INDUCTION

6. Connect a wire (or wire coil) to an ammeter. Wave a bar magnet close to but not touching the wire while observing the meter.

ANALYSIS

LAWS OF MAGNETISM

1. Which law of magnetism was illustrated by steps 1 and 2?

2. Which law of magnetism was illustrated by step 3?

3. State the law of magnetism that would require breaking the bar magnets.

MAPPING A STATIC FIELD

4. Draw the configuration of the magnetic lines of flux as revealed by the iron filings.

5. Why do the iron filings represent the magnetic lines of force?

MAPPING A DYNAMIC FIELD

6. What is represented by the changing of the direction of the compass needle?

7. Explain the reason for the change in the direction of the lines of force between steps 4 and 5.

8. Which of the Fleming Hand Rules is demonstrated by this experiment?

9. Draw in the appropriate compass needle directions, lines of force directions, and electron flow on Figure A for one direction flow and on Figure B for the other direction.

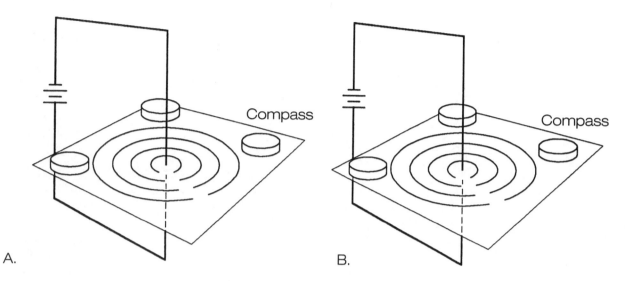

Compass

Compass

A.

B.

MAGNETIC INDUCTION

10. What effect does a moving magnetic field have on the current in a wire (or coil of wire)?

11. Explain (at the atomic level) how a moving magnetic field causes electrons to move along a wire thus producing current through magnetic induction.

12. Add arrows in the appropriate direction for the induced magnetic field in Figure C below.

Direction of Magnetic
Field Lines

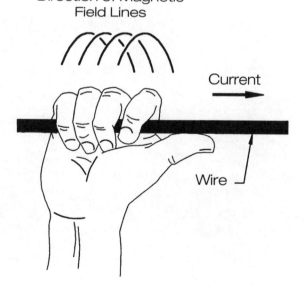

Current

Wire

C.

LABORATORY 4-2   ELECTROMAGNETIC INDUCTION

PURPOSE

Illustrate Faraday's Laws of electromagnetics.

MATERIALS

1. Helix coil of wire with few turns
2. Helix coil of wire with many turns
3. Moderately strong bar magnet
4. Strong bar magnet
5. Galvanometer (or ammeter)
6. Two connecting wires (preferably with alligator clips)

PROCEDURES

1. Use the wires to connect the ends of the helix coil with few turns to the meter. Record the approximate meter reading when the moderately strong bar magnet is moved at an average speed inside the coil. (If the coil is too small to accommodate the magnet, the magnet may be used to "stroke" the outside of the coil without touching the wires.)

2. Repeat step 1 with the strong bar magnet.

3. Repeat step 2 at high, moderate, and slow speed.

4. Repeat step 2 but with the magnet outside the coil moving at a 90° angle to the wire coils. Record the approximate meter reading at 90°, 45°, and parallel to the wire coils.

5. Repeat step 2 using the coil with few turns and again using the coil with many turns.

ANALYSIS

1. Complete the following data chart:

AMPERE READINGS									
strength		speed			angle			number of turns	
moderate	strong	slow	moderate	high	90°	45°	0°	few	many

2. Which of Faraday's Laws is demonstrated by procedure steps 1 and 2?

3. Which of Faraday's Laws is demonstrated by procedure step 3?

4. Which of Faraday's Laws is demonstrated by procedure step 4?

5. Which of Faraday's Laws is demonstrated by procedure step 5?

6. Label the arrows on the figure below to illustrate which indicates the direction of the magnetic field, current, and motion.

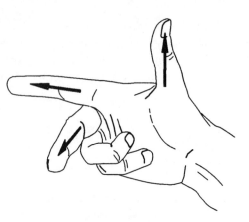

WORKSHEET 4–3   **GENERATORS, MOTORS, ALTERNATING AND DIRECT CURRENT**

PURPOSE

Explain the theory of generators and motors.

ACTIVITIES

1. An electric generator converts _____ energy into _____ energy.

2. In a generator, the conducting loops across which an emf is induced are called the _____.

3. A current that moves in one direction during part of the generating cycle and in a opposite direction during the remainder of the cycle is a(n) _____.

4. The output of a generator is increased by increasing the _____, or by increasing the number of _____ on the armature.

5. In using Fleming's Left Hand Generator Rule, when the thumb points in the direction the armature is moving and the index finger points in the direction of the magnetic flux, the middle finger indicates the direction of _____ flow.

6. A generator can supply _____ current, if its armature turns are connected to a commutator.

7. An electric motor converts _____ energy into _____ energy.

8. In using Fleming's Left Hand Motor Rule, when the thumb points in the direction the conductor is moving and the index finger points in the direction of the magnetic flux, the middle finger indicates the direction of _____ flow.

9. The synchronous motor is a constant _____ motor.

10. An induction motor uses a _____ to turn the rotor.

11. X-ray tubes use _____ motors to rotate the anode.

12. What are the essential components of an electric generator?

13. What are the essential components of an induction motor?

14. The following illustration represents the emf produced by an AC generator at various points as the armature coil wire rotates in the magnetic field.

   A. Draw arrows to show the direction of movement of the armature coil wire.

   B. Show conventional current flow through the armature coil wire at each point (A through I) in its rotation using the following method:

      1. Place a dot in the center of the conductor if the current flow is out of the page.
      2. Place a + in the center of the conductor if the current flow is into the page.
      3. Leave the conductor blank if there is no current flow.

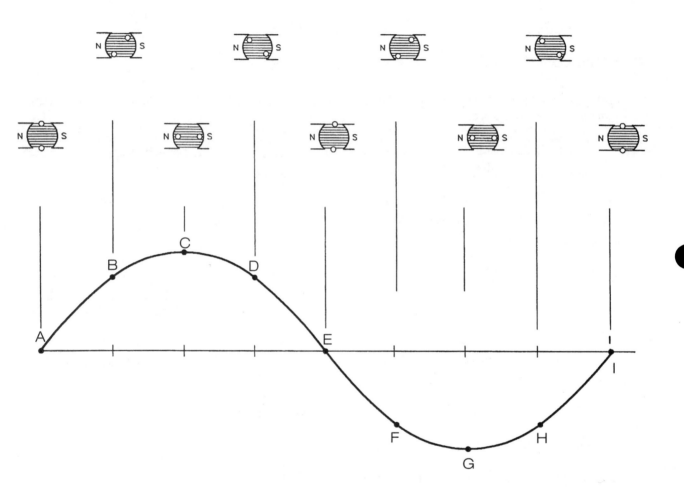

WORKSHEET 4–4   **TRANSFORMERS, AUTOTRANSFORMERS, AND CAPACITORS**

PURPOSE

Explain the effects of various types of transformers and capacitors on electrical current.

ACTIVITIES

1. Explain the basic concept of how a transformer uses induction to transform current.

2. Why won't a transformer function when supplied with direct current?

3. Explain in detail two of the three primary causes of transformer power loss.

4. What is the primary difference between a transformer and an autotransformer?

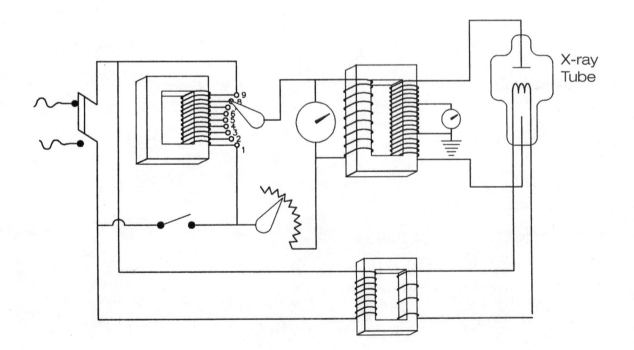

5. Label each transformer in the above drawing according to type (i.e., step-up, step-down, autotransformer). Place a "P" on the primary side and a "S" on the secondary side.

6. If a transformer is supplied with 200 volts to the primary coil, has 200 turns of wire on the primary coil and 40,000 turns of wire on the secondary coil, what will the voltage be in the secondary coil?

7. If a transformer has 1,600 turns of wire on the primary coil, 110 volts in the primary coil and 10 volts in the secondary coil, how many turns of wire must there be in the secondary coil?

8. How does a capacitor function?

PURPOSE

Analyze the direction of current flow for various rectification circuits.

ACTIVITIES

1. In the space above, draw a simple half-wave rectification circuit in which a single diode is used to protect the x-ray tube.

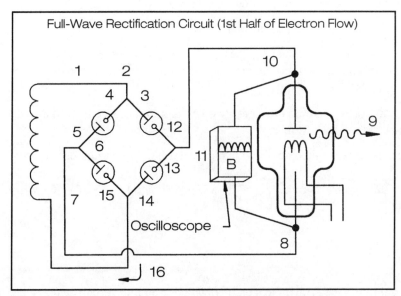

This figure may be replaced by an x-ray circuit simulator if one is available.

2. Observe the direction of the current at arrow 16 in the drawing. Draw in the appropriate arrows for 15 through 1 to show the direction of current for a full-wave rectification circuit.

3. Explain why the diode is placed on the cathode or anode side of a half-wave rectification circuit.

4. Number each of these descriptions to match the arrow in the drawing for #2.

_____ Conventional current flow is induced from the secondary coil of the high voltage step-up transformer.

_____ Current on this path reaches the heated cathode of valve tube III and easily jumps to the anode (thus never permitting enough charge to accumulate for the current at arrow 14 to jump across valve tube IV).

_____ Current on this path reaches the anode of valve tube I and distributes over the large unheated surface, attempting to build up enough charge to jump to the cathode.

_____ Current on this path reaches the anode of valve tube IV and distributes over the large unheated surface, attempting to build up enough charge to jump to the cathode.

_____ Current on this path moves without resistance toward the x-ray tube.

_____ Current reaches the x-ray tube heated cathode and jumps to the anode.

_____ Current on this path reaches the heated cathode of valve tube IV but cannot jump to the anode because the anode is still loaded with the charge moving at arrow 14. Because these are like charges they repel one another.

_____ X-rays are produced as a result of the current striking the anode.

_____ Current from the anode moves without resistance back toward the rectification circuit.

_____ Current reaches this junction and flows both ways.

_____ Current on this path reaches the heated cathode of valve tube II and easily jumps to the anode.

_____ Current reaches this junction and flows both ways.

_____ Current reaches this junction and flows both ways.

_____ Current on this path reaches the heated cathode of valve tube I but cannot jump to the anode because the anode is still loaded with the charge moving at arrow 5. Because these are like charges they repel one another.

_____ From this point on, current on this path moves without resistance toward the secondary coil of the high voltage step-up transformer.

_____ Current reaches the secondary coil of the high voltage step-up transformer, completing the circuit.

5. Would current flow through the x-ray tube, and if so would it be full- or half-wave rectified, if valve tube I burned out? II? III? IV?

6. Would current flow through the x-ray tube, and if so would it be full- or half-wave rectified, if valve tubes I and II burned out? I and III? I and IV? II and III? II and IV? III and IV?

7. Would current flow through the x-ray tube, and if so would it be full -or half-wave rectified, if valve tubes I, II, and III burned out? II, III, and IV?

WORKSHEET 5–1   **A BASIC X-RAY CIRCUIT**

PURPOSE

Construct a basic x-ray circuit from basic electrical devices.

ACTIVITIES

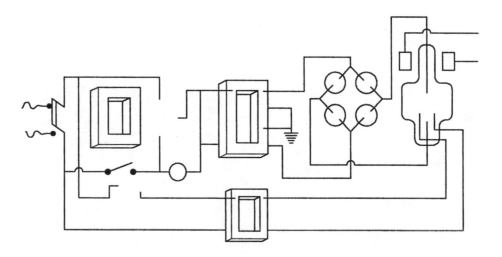

1. Draw in the appropriate coils for the 3 transformers to clearly indicate step-up, step-down, and autotransformers. Label each transformer's primary and secondary side as well as its type (i.e., step-up, etc.).

2. Draw in the mA control.

3. Draw in the diodes of the rectification circuit.

4. Draw in the anode and cathode of the x-ray tube.

5. Draw in a meter to measure the line voltage, amperage, and milliamperage.

6. Beginning at the main power breaker, draw arrows to indicate the flow of electrons through the complete circuit and draw a photon exiting the x-ray tube if your circuit would produce x-rays.

LABORATORY 5–2   GENERATORS

PURPOSE

Demonstrate the actual output waveform of an x-ray generator and explain the difference between different types of generators.

MATERIALS

1. Energized radiographic unit, single and/or three phase
2. X-ray output detector (some digital exposure timers and dosimeters are equipped with a BNC connector and can be used in this capacity)
3. Coaxial cable equipped with BNC connectors
4. Storage oscilloscope

SUGGESTED EXPOSURE FACTORS

100 mA, 0.5 sec, 80 kVp, 25" source to detector distance

PROCEDURES

1. Connect one end of the cable to the BNC output of the output detector and the other end to the BNC input on the oscilloscope.

2. Place detector on the radiographic table and center the x-ray tube to the detector. Turn on the oscilloscope and set the sensitivity level so that the oscilloscope is activated at the beginning of the x-ray waveform. The oscilloscope kilovoltage and time division controls should be set so that the output waveform covers the screen. Test exposures will have to be made to verify the appropriate oscilloscope settings. Refer to the oscilloscope operating manual or your instructor for help in obtaining the appropriate settings.

3. Expose the detector using the suggested exposure factors and view the output signal on the oscilloscope.

4. Draw the output waveform displayed.

5. Repeat the above steps using 90 kVp and using 70 kVp.

6. Draw the output waveforms displayed for kVp settings.

7. Repeat this activity using a generator with a different waveform.

RESULTS

1. Label the drawing of the output waveforms, to include the generator type, kVp, mA, and exposure time used.

ANALYSIS

1. Does the output waveform appear to match the theoretical waveform of the generator type used (see Chapter 5 of the textbook)? Explain your answer.

2. Compare the three output waveform drawings for a single generator type. Do they appear different? If so, how and why do they appear different? If not, should they have appeared different? How should they have appeared?

3. What diagnostic value does viewing output waveforms have in regard to generator condition?

4. Explain the output difference between a single-phase 2 pulse, a three-phase 6 pulse, and a three-phase 12 pulse generator.

5. Compare and contrast high frequency and three-phase 12 pulse generators with respect to their output and design.

6. Explain the difference between a falling load and constant potential generator.

WORKSHEET 6-1   X-RAY TUBES

PURPOSE

Describe the basic components and operation of a modern x-ray tube.

MATERIALS

Various x-ray tubes

ACTIVITIES

1. Label the components of the x-ray tube in the drawing below.

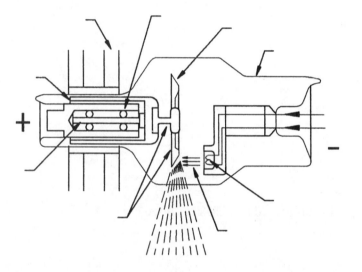

2.   Examine the various x-ray tubes.

    a.   Spin the anode and describe the sound (rough, smooth, etc.).

    b.   Using a protractor, determine the angle of the anode(s) and record them.

    c.   Identify the number of filaments in the cathode assembly for each tube.

    d.   Describe any signs of tube wear or failure.

3.   What is thermionic emission?

4. What is the function of the focusing cup?

5. What is the advantage of a rotating anode over a stationary anode?

6. Explain the line-focus principle.

7. How does the target angle affect the size of the effective focal spot? Draw a diagram to illustrate this concept.

8. Describe the anode heel effect.

9. How is the anode heel effect influenced by field size? distance?

WORKSHEET 6–2   **RATING CHARTS AND COOLING CHARTS**

PURPOSE

Determine safe tube exposures using a rating chart and cooling chart.

ACTIVITIES

1. Based on the tube rating chart below, circle the exposures that would be safe.

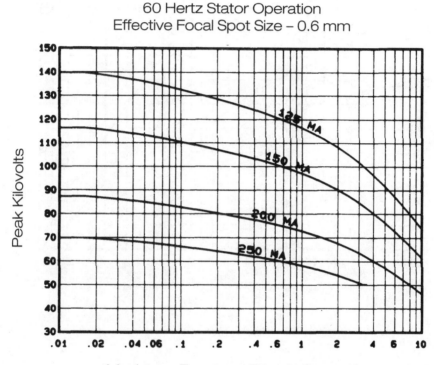

60 Hertz Stator Operation
Effective Focal Spot Size – 0.6 mm

Peak Kilovolts

Maximum Exposure Time In Seconds

Courtesy of Varian EIMAC.

   a.   125 mA, 0.4 sec, 120 kVp

   b.   150 mA, 0.5 sec, 80 kVp

   c.   150 mA, 2 sec, 100 kVp

   d.   200 mA, 0.08 sec, 90 kVp

e.   200 mA, 0.1 sec, 70 kVp

   f.   200 mA, 0.6 sec, 80 kVp

   g.   250 mA, 0.2 sec, 70 kVp

   h.   250 mA, 2 sec, 50 kVp

2.   Based on the tube rating chart below, circle the exposures that would be safe.

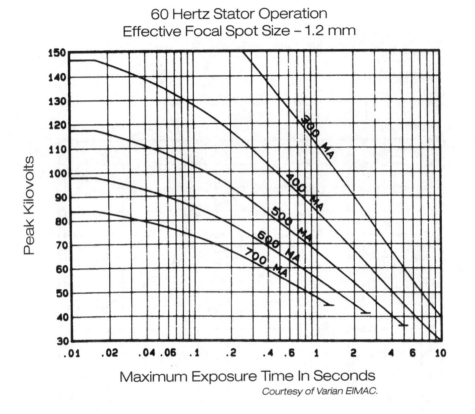

60 Hertz Stator Operation
Effective Focal Spot Size – 1.2 mm

Peak Kilovolts

Maximum Exposure Time In Seconds

Courtesy of Varian EIMAC.

   a.   300 mA, 0.5 sec, 110 kVp

   b.   400 mA, 0.3 sec, 100 kVp

   c.   400 mA, 1 sec, 80 kVp

   d.   500 mA, 0.2 sec, 60 kVp

   e.   500 mA, 2 sec, 70 kVp

   f.   600 mA, 0.04 sec, 90 kVp

   g.   600 mA, 0.1 sec, 90 kVp

   h.   700 mA, 0.2 sec, 70 kVp

3. Calculate the heat units generated for the following exposures:

Single-phase, full-wave unit

a. 100 mA, 0.05 sec, 60 kVp

b. 300 mA, 0.4 sec, 85 kVp

Three-phase, 6 pulse unit

c. 200 mA, 0.25 sec, 72 kVp

d. 600 mA, 0.6 sec, 88 kVp

Three-phase, 12 pulse unit

e. 400 mA, 0.33 sec, 90 kVp

f. 1,000 mA, 0.02 sec, 120 kVp

Use the anode cooling chart below to answer the following questions.

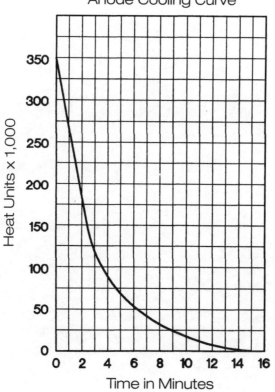

Anode Cooling Curve

4. Calculate the length of time necessary for the anode to cool to 25,000 heat units after 12 exposures of 600 mA, 0.2 sec, at 70 kVp.

5. Calculate the length of time necessary for the anode to cool completely after 10 exposures of 1,000 mA, 0.05 sec, at 80 kVp.

WORKSHEET 7–1   **X-RAY PRODUCTION**

PURPOSE

Explain the process of x-ray production.

ACTIVITIES

1.   What conditions are necessary for the production of x-rays?

2.   What percentage of the kinetic energy of the electrons is converted to x-rays? What happens to the rest of the energy?

3.   What are the two target interactions that can produce x-rays?

4. Study the illustration below.

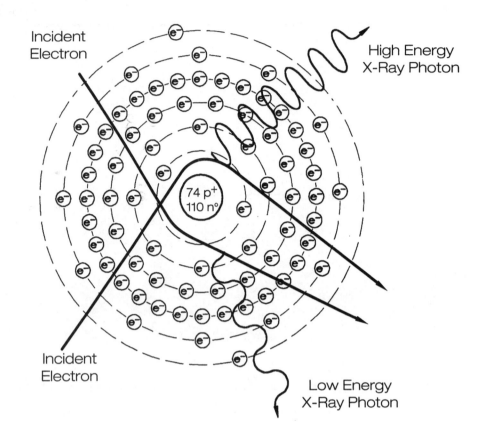

a. What interaction is illustrated above?

b. What determines the energy of the photon produced during this interaction?

5.   Study the illustration below.

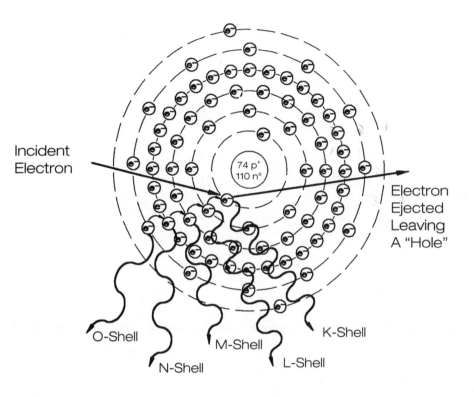

a.   What interaction is illustrated above?

b.   What determines the energy of the photon produced during this interaction?

6.   What is meant by a characteristic cascade?

7. What is the K-shell binding energy for the following elements?

   a. hydrogen

   b. calcium

   c. iodine

   d. barium

   e. tungsten

   f. lead

8. What is meant by kilovoltage peak?

9. What is the relationship between the kilovoltage peak and the average energy (keV) of the photons in the primary beam?

LABORATORY 8–1 _____ **USING DOSIMETRY EQUIPMENT**

PURPOSE

Use basic ionizing radiation dosimetry equipment.

MATERIALS

1. Energized radiographic unit
2. Abdomen phantom
3. Dosimeter
4. Ring stand

PROCEDURES

1. Position the abdomen phantom on the x-ray table. Use the ring stand to center the dosimeter directly over the sacrum at the point where the beam will enter the phantom.

2. Follow the instructions with the dosimetry equipment to record three exposures to the phantom.

RESULTS

1. Record the three exposures.

ANALYSIS

1. How close to one another were the three exposures?

2. What was the average exposure?

3. If exposures of 65 mR, 62 mR, and 131 mR were recorded, it would be advisable to perform three additional exposures. If the second set of exposures were 62 mR, 66 mR, and 65 mR, what would you record as the average exposure?

4.   Why is it advised that the average of three exposures be used for all dosimetry measurements?

LABORATORY 9-1   BASIC RADIATION PROTECTION, DETECTION, AND MEASUREMENT

PURPOSE

Introduce commonly used radiation protection techniques and devices and demonstrate their effectiveness in reducing exposure to patient and operator.

MATERIALS

1. Energized radiographic unit (assumed to include about 2.5 mm/Al Eq filtration)
2. Abdomen phantom
3. Dosimeter
4. Flat contact gonad shields
5. Ring stand

PROCEDURES

1. Become familiar with the common radiation protection devices and techniques as introduced by your instructor.

2. Set up the x-ray tube and phantom as if to do an AP pelvis using a 40" SID. Raise the phantom with sponges or sheets to create a tunnel large enough to accommodate the dosimeter ion chamber underneath the phantom.

   A. SOMATIC EXPOSURE – Entrance Skin Exposure (ESE)

      1. Effect of Filtration

         a. Center the ionization chamber on the anterior surface of the pelvis. Using a 14" x 17" field size, 70 kVp, and 60 mAs, expose and record ESE in mR on table A.

         b. Center the ionization chamber on the posterior surface of the pelvis. Using a 14" x 17" field size, 70 kVp, and 60 mAs, expose and record exit exposure in mR on table A.

         c. Repeat 1a and 1b with 1 mm aluminum added to the primary beam for a total of about 3.5 mm Al.

         d. Repeat 1a and 1b with about 1 mm/Al filtration removed for a total of about 1.5 mm Al.

      2. Effect of kVp

         a. Repeat 1a and 1b but change technique to 60 kVp and 120 mAs. (This new technique is a result of using the 15% rule in order to increase the contrast.)

         b. Repeat 1a and 1b but change technique to 80 kVp and 30 mAs. (This new technique is a result of using the 15% rule in order to decrease the contrast.)

B. GONAD EXPOSURE (MALE)

1. Use the ring stand to place the ionization chamber at the approximate location of the testes. Collimate the beam so the testes would be included in the beam. Using 70 kVp and 60 mAs, expose and record exposure in mR on table B.

2. Repeat B1 using a flat gonad shield placed over the area of the testes.

3. Repeat B1 with the beam collimated to the edge of the area of the testes. Do not use a shield.

4. Repeat B3 using a flat gonad shield placed over the area of the testes.

5. Repeat B1 using a collimated beam that excludes the area of the testes by 5 cm or more. Do not use the shield.

RESULTS

TABLE A

	kVp	mAs	SID	Total Filtration (Al Eq)	ESE (mR)	Exit Exposure (mR)
	70	60	40"	2.5 mm Al		
Effect of Filtration	70	60	40"	3.5 mm Al		
	70	60	40"	1.5 mm Al		
Effect of kVp	60	120	40"	2.5 mm Al		
	80	30	40"	2.5 mm Al		

TABLE B

	EXPOSURE TO TESTES (mR)	
BEAM COLLIMATION	No Shield	Shield
Include Testes		
Exclude Testes		
Exclude Testes by 5 cm		xxxxxxxxxxxxxxxxxx

ANALYSIS

1. Which method(s) investigated reduced the ESE's to the pelvis?

2. Which method had the greatest effect on reducing the ESE's? Why do you think this method is so effective in reducing exposure?

3. Name two other possible methods that could be utilized in reducing the exposure to the patient.

4. List in order the protective methods used in the demonstration according to the gonad exposure received. List the least protective first. Briefly, why do you believe the list is arranged as it is?

5. Why is gonad shielding so important? Why are the male gonads more sensitive to exposure than the female gonads?

LABORATORY 10-1

EFFECTS OF FILTRATION

PURPOSE

Demonstrate the effect of filtration on x-ray emission.

MATERIALS

1. Energized radiographic unit
2. Aluminum filters (0.25, 0.5, 1.0, 2.0 mm Al)
3. Dosimeter

SUGGESTED EXPOSURE FACTORS

100 mAs for three-phase generators, 200 mAs for single-phase generators, 60 kVp, 40" SID

PROCEDURES

1. Center the dosimeter to the center of the x-ray field.

2. Direct the central ray perpendicular to the center of the dosimeter and collimate to a 4" x 4" field size.

3. Remove all added filtration from the x-ray tube. If this is not possible, the radiographic unit may be used as it is normally filtered. Expose the dosimeter.

4. Record the exposure received by the dosimeter as no aluminum added.

5. Add a 0.25 mm aluminum filter to the primary beam. The aluminum filters may be sequentially taped to the face of the collimator. Expose the dosimeter using the same exposure factors and record the exposure.

6. Add an additional 0.5 mm aluminum filter and repeat as above. Follow the same procedures for 1.0 mm Al and 2.0 mm Al.

7. Reduce the mAs by 50% and repeat steps 1–8 using 90 kVp.

RESULTS

Dosimeter readings

Filtration	60 kVp	90 kVp
no aluminum added	_____mR	_____mR
0.25 mm aluminum	_____mR	_____mR
0.5 mm aluminum	_____mR	_____mR
1.0 mm aluminum	_____mR	_____mR
2.0 mm aluminum	_____mR	_____mR

ANALYSIS

1. Based on the results obtained, what is the effect of adding filtration on x-ray emission? What would be the effect on radiographic density?

2. What is the purpose of filtering the radiographic beam?

3. What is the difference between inherent, added, and total filtration?

4. What is the total filtration requirement for x-ray tubes that operate at 70 kVp and above?

LABORATORY 10–2   HALF-VALUE LAYER DETERMINATION

PURPOSE

To calculate the half-value layer of a given x-ray unit.

MATERIALS

1. Energized radiographic unit
2. 4 Aluminum attenuators (1.0 mm Al sheets)
3. Dosimeter

SUGGESTED EXPOSURE FACTORS

100 mAs for three-phase generators, 200 mAs for single-phase generators, 80 kVp, 40" SID

PROCEDURES

1. Center the dosimeter ionization chamber to the center of the x-ray field. Collimate to a 4" x 4" field size.

2. Expose the dosimeter using the suggested exposure factors and record the exposure received by the dosimeter.

3. Form a shelf below the collimator by loosely taping a 1 mm Al attenuator to the collimator housing. This shelf will be used to hold additional Al attenuators. **NOTE: Make sure the Al attenuator intercepts the entire field of the collimator light.** Repeat step 2.

4. In sequence, add three 1.0 mm Al attenuators to the shelf, repeating step 2 after adding each one.

RESULTS

Dosimeter readings

Filtration	80 kVp
no aluminum added	_____mR
1 mm aluminum added	_____mR
2 mm aluminum added	_____mR
3 mm aluminum added	_____mR
4 mm aluminum added	_____mR

ANALYSIS

1. Plot calculated mR values vs. total thickness of the Al attenuators added to the x-ray beam, on semi-Log graph paper. Draw a straight line through plotted data points. The thickness of added Al attenuators that reduces the exposure output with 0 mm Al added by one half is the measured half-value layer. What is the measured half-value layer?

2. A single-phase x-ray tube with a total filtration of 2.5 mm Al/Eq should produce an x-ray beam with a half-value layer of 2.4 mm Al using 80 kVp. A three-phase x-ray tube with a total filtration of 2.5 mm Al/Eq should produce an x-ray beam with a half-value layer of 2.7 mm Al using 80 kVp. Explain why the recommended half-value layers are different.

3. What are some of the possible causes for the HVL being less than that recommended? What is/are the practical implication(s) of this situation?

4. What are some of the possible causes for the HVL being excessively large in comparison to the recommended value? What is/are the practical implication(s) of this situation?

5. Define half-value layer.

WORKSHEET 11-1   CALCULATING PRIME FACTORS

PURPOSE

Perform calculations to adjust the various prime factors.

ACTIVITIES

1. Given the following mA and exposure times, calculate the mAs.

	mA	time		mAs
a.	200	1/40	=	_____
b.	400	3/10	=	_____
c.	300	3/5	=	_____
d.	100	1/20	=	_____
e.	600	1/4	=	_____
f.	100	.05	=	_____
g.	400	.017	=	_____
h.	300	.20	=	_____
i.	200	.33	=	_____
j.	1,000	.006	=	_____

2. Given the following mAs and mA values, calculate the exposure time.

	mA	time		mAs
a.	100	_____	=	75
b.	300	_____	=	120
c.	200	_____	=	5
d.	600	_____	=	15
e.	400	_____	=	80

51

3. Given the following mAs and exposure time values, calculate the mA.

	mA	time		mAs
a.	____	.03	=	30
b.	____	.05	=	35
c.	____	.7	=	210
d.	____	1/4	=	75
e.	____	1/10	=	60

4. Using the inverse square law, calculate the new exposure rate when the distance is changed.

a. 36 inch SID   40 inch SID
   250 mR   ____mR

b. 28 inch SID   42 inch SID
   175 mR   ____mR

c. 36 inch SID   72 inch SID
   100 mR   ____mR

d. 40 inch SID   72 inch SID
   125 mR   ____mR

e. 40 inch SID   56 inch SID
   80 mR   ____mR

5. Using the density maintenance formula, calculate the missing factor.

a. 40 inch SID   72 inch SID
   40 mAs   ____mAs

b. 72 inch SID   36 inch SID
   75 mAs   ____mAs

c. 40 inch SID   56 inch SID
   160 mAs   ____ mAs

d. 40 inch SID   ____SID
   12 mAs   27 mAs

e. 72 inch SID   ____SID
   20 mAs   10 mAs

6. Using the 15% rule, calculate the kVp that will produce the same density as the original set of factors.

a. 150 mAs   300 mAs
   60 kVp   ____kVp

b. 25 mAs   50 mAs
   80 kVp   ____kVp

c. 60 mAs   120 mAs
   75 kVp   ____kVp

d. 200 mAs   100 mAs
   90 kVp   ____ kVp

e. 10 mAs   5 mAs
   50 kVp   ____kVp

LABORATORY 11–2   EFFECT OF mAs, kVp, AND SID ON X-RAY EMISSION

PURPOSE

Demonstrate the effect of mAs, kVp, and SID on x-ray emission.

MATERIALS

1. Energized radiographic unit
2. Dosimeter

SUGGESTED EXPOSURE FACTORS

100 mA, 0.1 sec, 10 mAs, 50 kVp, 36" SID

PROCEDURES

1. Place the dosimeter ion chamber in the center of the x-ray beam.

2. Direct the central ray perpendicular to the center of the ion chamber and collimate to a 5" x 5" field size.

3. Expose the ion chamber and record the results.

mAs/X-RAY EMISSION

4. Repeat steps 1–3, changing the suggested factors to 20 mAs.

5. Repeat steps 1–3, changing the suggested factors to 30 mAs.

kVp/X-RAY EMISSION

6. Repeat steps 1–3, changing the suggested factors to 60 kVp.

7. Repeat steps 1–3, changing the suggested factors to 70 kVp.

SID/X-RAY EMISSION

8. Repeat steps 1–3, changing the suggested factors to 56" SID.

9. Repeat steps 1–3, changing the suggested exposure factors to 72" SID.

RESULTS

1. Record the dosimeter readings:

    Initial exposure _____

    mAs/X-RAY EMISSION

        20 mAs _____   30 mAs _____

    kVp/X-RAY EMISSION

        60 kVp _____   70 kVp _____

    SID/X-RAY EMISSION

        56" SID _____   72" SID _____

ANALYSIS

mAs/X-RAY EMISSION

1. What effect does increasing mAs have on the exposure?

2. What is the specific relationship between mAs and x-ray emission?

kVp/X-RAY EMISSION

3. What effect does increasing kVp have on exposure?

4. What is the specific relationship between kVp and x-ray emission?

SID/X-RAY EMISSION

5. What effect does increasing SID have on x-ray exposure?

6. What is the specific relationship between SID and x-ray emission?

WORKSHEET 12–1   **X-RAY INTERACTIONS**

PURPOSE

Explain the interactions between x-rays and matter.

ACTIVITIES

1.   Draw a diagram to illustrate the photoelectric interaction between x-ray and matter.

2.   How is secondary radiation produced?

3.   Draw a diagram to illustrate the Compton interaction between x-ray and matter.

4.   How is scatter radiation produced?

5.   What is the predominant interaction in the diagnostic x-ray range?

6.   What is the relationship of kVp to the incidence of x-ray interaction?

7.   How does kVp affect the number of photoelectric versus Compton interactions?

8.   How does scatter radiation affect image contrast?

9.   Explain the process of coherent scattering.

LABORATORY 13-1   ESTIMATING PATIENT ENTRANCE SKIN EXPOSURE

PURPOSE

Estimate entrance skin exposure (ESE) for various radiographic projections.

MATERIALS

1. Energized radiographic unit
2. Digital dosimeter
3. Technique chart

PROCEDURES

1. Obtain a reliable technique chart (ideally one that is used in clinical practice) and using the techniques from the chart, calculate the ESE values for a 23 cm PA chest, 15 cm lateral skull, 23 cm AP abdomen, 23 cm AP L–Spine, and a 13 cm AP C–Spine according to the following steps:

2. Set the tube SID at the appropriate distance for the projection, place the dosimeter's ion chamber detector on the radiographic table, center, and collimate the beam to the appropriate part size. Set the exposure factors according to the chart, turn on the digital dosimeter unit, select the single-dose mode, and follow the manufacturer's instructions, record an exposure.

3. Determine the thickness of the detector and the distance from the Bucky tray to the table top (part film distance) in cm. Use these figures to determine the source to skin distance (SSD) and the source to detector distance (SDD).

4. Use the inverse square law to determine the ESE delivered to the body part.

$$\frac{\text{dosimeter exposure reading (mR)}}{\text{ESE (mR)}} = \frac{\text{SSD}^2}{\text{SDD}^2}$$

<u>Bucky techniques</u>

SSD = SID − (part thickness + part film distance)

SDD = SID − (detector thickness + part film distance)

<u>Table techniques</u>

SSD = SID − part thickness

SDD = SID − detector thickness

RESULTS

1.   Record your data below

	Dosimeter Exposure (mR)	SSD (cm)	SDD (cm)	ESE (mR)
AP chest	_____	_____	_____	_____
Lateral skull	_____	_____	_____	_____
AP abdomen	_____	_____	_____	_____
AP C–Spine	_____	_____	_____	_____
AP L–Spine	_____	_____	_____	_____

ANALYSIS

1.   What is the ESE for the five projections?

2.   Compare your ESE results with the Conference of Radiation Control Program Directors Average Patient Exposure Guides in the textbook.

3.   Describe three ways that ESE can be reduced.

4.   What correlations can be drawn about ESE and organ dose?

LABORATORY 14–1 ━━━━━━━━━━━━━━━━━━━━━━━━━━━━ THINKING THREE-DIMENSIONALLY

PURPOSE

Illustrate the importance of multiple projections in perceiving the radiographic image as representation of a three-dimensional object.

MATERIALS

1. Energized radiographic unit
2. Chest phantom with hollow lungfields is preferred although a solid chest, abdomen, or pelvis phantom can be substituted
3. 14" x 17" cassette with film
4. Dosimeter
5. Film processor

SUGGESTED EXPOSURE FACTORS

Chest: 400 RS, 4 mAs, 80 kVp, 72" SID, non grid
Abdomen: 400 RS, 20 mAs, 80 kVp, 40" SID, 8:1 Bucky grid

PROCEDURES

1. The instructor prepares the phantom by taping several artifacts (keys, hairpins, paper clips, etc.) onto the phantom—at least one each on the surface located anterior, posterior, right lateral, left lateral, and opposite obliques (i.e., right posterior and left anterior surfaces). When a hollow chest phantom can be used, half the artifacts should be inside the chest wall and half outside. Each artifact must be located at a separate superior-inferior location so that no two artifacts will be superimposed on AP, oblique, or lateral radiographs. The prepared phantom is then covered with a patient gown to hide artifact locations from students.

2. Chest phantom: Place the phantom vertically on the table top and center it to a loaded cassette held vertical in a cassette holder.

   Abdomen/pelvis phantom: Place the phantom recumbent on the table and center it to a loaded cassette in the Bucky tray.

3. Direct the central ray perpendicular to the center of the film, position the phantom for an AP position, and collimate to the part.

4. Expose and process the film. Label the film by position.

5. Repeat steps 2–4 for a left lateral, LPO, and RPO position.

RESULTS

1. Use a marker to number each artifact on all 4 films (i.e., label the first artifact #1 on the AP, lateral, and both oblique films, the second artifact #2 on each film, etc.).

ANALYSIS

1. Give the precise location of each artifact on the phantom. For example, specify location as to anterior, posterior, right or left lateral, RPO, LPO, LAO, RAO surface. For a hollow chest phantom, specify whether the artifact is located inside or outside the chest wall.

2. Give the minimum number of projections that are necessary to locate each artifact and explain why fewer projections would not define each location.

LABORATORY 15–1   **BEAM RESTRICTION**

PURPOSE

Demonstrate the effects of beam restriction on radiographic image quality.

MATERIALS

1. Energized radiographic unit
2. Automatic film processor
3. Phantom knee
4. 10" x 12" cassettes with film
5. 2 water-filled plastic gallon jugs

SUGGESTED EXPOSURE FACTORS

400 RS, 100 mA, 0.05 sec, 70 kVp, 40" SID, non grid

PROCEDURES

1. Make two exposures of the knee in a PA position using table top procedure and two 10" x 12" cassettes. Two water-filled jugs will be used to simulate extra tissue.

2. Center the cassette lengthwise to the table top. Center the knee to the cassette and place the water jugs on both sides. Center to the knee and open collimators to include as much of the water jugs as possible and expose.

3. Repeat step 2, but collimate the beam closely to include just the knee.

4. Process films.

RESULTS

1. Review the radiographs with respect to radiographic density and contrast differences exhibited.

ANALYSIS

1. Which radiograph demonstrates the best image quality? Why?

2.   What is/are the factor(s) that caused the change in the quality of the two images?

3.   What patient-related factors contribute to the production of scatter radiation?

4.   What x-ray beam related factors contribute to the production of scatter radiation?

5.   Describe four different devices that are used in diagnostic radiology for beam restriction.

LABORATORY 16–1   EFFECT OF SUBJECT ON ATTENUATION AND SCATTER

PURPOSE

Demonstrate the effect of subject thickness on attenuation and scatter of the primary x-ray beam.

MATERIALS

1. Energized radiographic unit
2. Automatic film processor
3. Abdomen phantom
4. 14" x 17" radiographic cassettes with film
5. 14" x 17" wire mesh test tool
6. Cassette holder
7. Dosimeter

SUGGESTED EXPOSURE FACTORS

20 mAs, 95 kVp, 40" SID, non grid

PROCEDURES

1. Place the abdomen phantom in an AP position on sponges or sheets high enough to create a tunnel of sufficient height to permit the placement of the dosimeter chamber underneath the phantom. Center the phantom to the table top with the central ray perpendicular to the level of the iliac crest and collimate to the abdomen. Place the dosimeter detector on the anterior surface of the abdomen at the location of the CR and expose. Record the dosimeter reading in mR as the entrance exposure.

2. Repeat step 1, but place the dosimeter detector at the posterior surface of the phantom at the location of the CR. Record the dosimeter reading in mR as the exit exposure.

3. Place the wire mesh test tool on top of a loaded 14" x 17" cassette. Secure both crosswise in a vertical position using a cassette holder as shown below. Position the cassette holder so that the cassette is approximately one inch from the lateral edge of the phantom and centered to the level of the iliac crest. Using a perpendicular CR, center the tube to the level of the iliac crest and collimate the beam to the abdomen. The primary beam should not include any portion of the vertical cassette. Expose the phantom using the technique in step 1 and process the film.

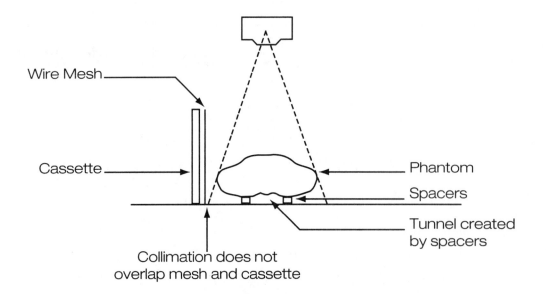

Wire Mesh

Cassette

Collimation does not
overlap mesh and cassette

Phantom

Spacers

Tunnel created
by spacers

4. Position the phantom for a lateral abdomen. Center a perpendicular CR to the level of the iliac crest and collimate to the phantom, using a 40" SID. Place the dosimeter detector on the superior lateral surface of the phantom at the location of the CR. Expose using 5 mAs at 95 kVp. Record the dosimeter reading in mR as the
entrance exposure.

5. Repeat step 4, but place the dosimeter detector at the inferior lateral surface of the phantom at the location of
the CR. Record the dosimeter reading in mR as the exit exposure.

6. Place the wire mesh test tool on top of a loaded 14" x 17" cassette. Secure both crosswise in a vertical position
using a cassette holder. Position the cassette holder so that the cassette is approximately one inch from the
posterior surface of the phantom and centered to the level of the iliac crest. Using a perpendicular CR, center
it to the level of the iliac crest and collimate the beam to the phantom. The primary beam should not include
the vertical cassette. Expose the phantom using the technique in step 4 and process the film.

7. Use a densitometer to measure the optical density at the center of the bottom, middle, and top thirds of both
radiographs. Record the readings.

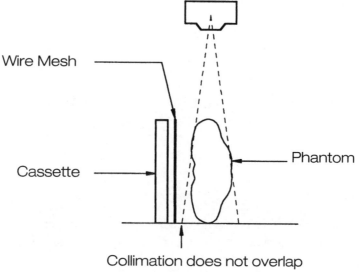

Wire Mesh

Cassette

Phantom

Collimation does not overlap
mesh and cassette

RESULTS

<u>ATTENUATION</u>

Projection	Part Thickness	Entrance Exposure (mR)	Exit Exposure (mR)
AP Abdomen	_____	_____	_____
Lat Abdomen	_____	_____	_____

<u>SCATTER</u>

Projection	Part Thickness	OD of Film Bottom 1/3	Middle 1/3	Top 1/3
AP Abdomen	_____	_____	_____	_____
Lateral Abdomen	_____	_____	_____	_____

ANALYSIS

1. Were the entrance exposures similar or different for the AP and lateral abdomen? Why?

2. Were the exit exposures similar or different for the AP and lateral abdomen? Why?

3. Which radiograph showed the greatest amount of radiographic density? Why?

4. Were you able to demonstrate a difference between the radiographic densities produced on the bottom, middle, and top thirds of the AP abdomen radiograph? If so, how would you explain this?

5. Were you able to demonstrate a difference between the radiographic densities produced on the bottom, middle, and top thirds of the lateral abdomen radiograph? If so, how would you explain this?

6. What happens to the quality and quantity of the beam as it passes from entrance to exit through the patient? How were these effects demonstrated on the radiographs you produced as part of this lab?

7. List all the subject-related factors that would have a bearing on attenuation and scatter of the beam.

8. Are there factors besides the subject that affect the attenuation and scatter of the beam? Explain.

WORSHEET 17-1   **THE EFFECT OF PATHOLOGY ON IMAGE QUALITY**

PURPOSE

Illustrate the effect of pathology on image quality.

MATERIALS

Radiographs demonstrating:

Chest   Abdomen

congestive heart failure   ascites
emphysema   bowel obstruction
pleural effusion
pneumonia   Extremities/Skull
pneumothorax
tuberculosis   active osteomyelitis
                                              degenerative arthritis
                                              osteoporosis
                                              Paget's disease

ACTIVITIES

1.   Based on a review of the radiographs, which of the images demonstrates an increased attenuation (additive) condition?

2.   What causes a pathologic condition to result in an increased attenuation of the x-ray beam?

3. Based on a review of the radiographs, which of the images demonstrates a decreased attenuation (destructive) condition?

4. What causes a pathologic condition to result in a decreased attenuation of the x-ray beam?

5. Based on a review of the radiographs, which images required an adjustment from normal technical factors used for the procedure?

6. What technical factor adjustments are recommended for additive conditions? for destructive conditions?

LABORATORY 18-1   **GRID COMPARISONS AND CONVERSIONS**

PURPOSE

Demonstrate the use of grid conversion factors.

MATERIALS

1. Energized radiographic unit
2. Automatic film processor
3. 8:1 and 12:1 radiographic grids
4. Abdomen phantom
5. Cassettes with film
6. Step wedge (penetrometer)
7. Densitometer

SUGGESTED EXPOSURE FACTORS

400 RS, 200 mA, 0.03 sec, 75 kVp, 40" SID, non grid

PROCEDURES

1. Center the abdomen phantom to the cassette on the table top. Place the step wedge beside the phantom on the cassette. Direct the central ray perpendicular to the center of the cassette and collimate to the edges.

2. Use the suggested factors to expose the film, process, and label it #1. Use a densitometer to measure the OD of step 5. If it is not 1.2 ± 0.2, adjust the mAs and re-expose.

3. Repeat step 1 using an 8:1 ratio grid. Expose the film using the appropriate grid conversion factor, process, and label it #2. If it is not 1.2 ± 0.2, adjust the mAs and re-expose.

4. Repeat step 1 using a 12:1 ratio grid. Expose the film using the appropriate grid conversion factor, process, and label it #3. If it is not 1.2 ± 0.2, adjust the mAs and re-expose.

5. Use a densitometer to measure the OD (optical density) of step 5 on the step wedge for all the films and record the readings in the results section.

RESULTS

1. Review the three radiographs in terms of their radiographic density.

   Step 5 Optical Density (OD)

   Radiograph #1 _____

   Radiograph #2 _____

   Radiograph #3 _____

ANALYSIS

1. When is it necessary to use a radiographic grid for an examination?

2. Describe the appearance of radiographs 1, 2, and 3. Which one(s) more closely approximate(s) a quality image? Why?

3. Where were the radiographic densities of the three images the same? If they were not, were the differences significant? Explain.

4. Based on your data, what conclusions can you draw about the effect of grids and grid ratios on conversion factors?

5. What factors or influences contribute to the decrease or increase of image quality in each of the radiographs?

6. Based on the procedure, what is the importance of a radiographic grid?

LABORATORY 18-2 GRID ERRORS

PURPOSE

Demonstrate the effects of the common errors accompanying the use of radiographic grids.

MATERIALS

1. Energized radiographic unit
2. Automatic film processor
3. 12:1 80 line/inch linear focused grid
4. Cassettes with film
5. Skull phantom

SUGGESTED EXPOSURE FACTORS

400 RS, 50 mA, 0.15 sec, 80 kVp, 40" SID, 12:1 stationary grid

PROCEDURES

1. Center a 10" x 12" stationary linear focused grid on a 10" x 12" loaded cassette placed crosswise in the center of a radiographic table. Position the phantom skull for a lateral projection, making sure the perpendicular CR is directed to the center of the grid. Expose using the suggested exposure factors.

2. Process the film and label it radiograph #1.

3. Repeat step 1, but move the perpendicular CR approximately 3" toward the top of the skull so that it is off center of grid center line. Open collimator sufficiently to expose the entire cassette. Process the film and label it radiograph #2.

4. Repeat step 1, but angle the CR caudally 15 degrees across the grid's center line with it centered to the grid. Adjust the SID to compensate for the angulation and open collimator sufficiently to expose the entire cassette. Process the film and label it radiograph #3.

5. Repeat step 1, but elevate the side of the cassette under the chin 15 degrees from the plane of the table using a positioning sponge. Adjust the phantom skull to maintain its lateral position. Process the film and label it radiograph #4.

6. Repeat step 1, but turn the grid upside down. Make sure the CR is centered to the grid. Process the film and label it radiograph #5.

7. Repeat step 1, but use a 50" SID. Process the film and label it radiograph #6.

8. Repeat step 1, but use a 30" SID. Process the film and label it radiograph #7.

RESULTS

1. Using radiograph #1 as the standard for comparison, review the six radiographs with respect to image quality.

ANALYSIS

1. Describe radiographs 2 through 7 with respect to their image quality.

2. Which grid error(s) had the worst effect on the image quality? Explain the reason for this occurring.

3. Which grid error(s) had the least effect on the image quality? Explain the reason for this occurring.

4. Would you expect the results to be more or less severe with a lower ratio grid? Justify your answer.

5. Based on the results of the experiment, state at least four rules that should be followed when using linear focused grids.

LABORATORY 18-3   THE AIR GAP TECHNIQUE

PURPOSE

Demonstrate the effects of the air gap technique on radiographic image quality.

MATERIALS

1. Energized radiographic unit
2. Automatic film processor
3. Skull phantom
4. 10" x 12" cassettes with film
5. Densitometer

SUGGESTED EXPOSURE FACTORS

400 RS, 100 mA, .04 sec, 80 kVp, 40" SID, non grid

PROCEDURES

1. Position the skull phantom for a lateral projection using a 10" x 12" cassette crosswise on the tabletop. Center and collimate the beam to the cassette. Expose the film using the suggested exposure factors, process, and label it #1.

2. Repeat step 1 with the skull elevated 7" above the cassette. Use positioning sponges or other appropriate means to achieve this effect. Expose, process the film, and label it #2.

3. Measure and record the optical density of the sella turcica for each radiograph using a densitometer.

RESULTS

1. Visually review and compare the two radiographs with regard to their image quality.

2. Record the optical density measurements of the sella turcica.

                                    Optical Density

Skull in contact with cassette (#1)   _____

Skull with 7" air gap (#2)   _____

ANALYSIS

1. Was there a difference in the optical densities of the sella turcica on the two radiographs? If so, was the difference significant? Explain the reason for the difference.

2. Describe any other differences between the images that are apparent and explain the reason(s) for the difference(s).

3. Give at least two clinical applications for the air gap technique and explain the rationale for its use in each case.

WORKSHEET 19–1   **LATENT IMAGE FORMATION**

PURPOSE

Describe latent image formation.

ACTIVITIES

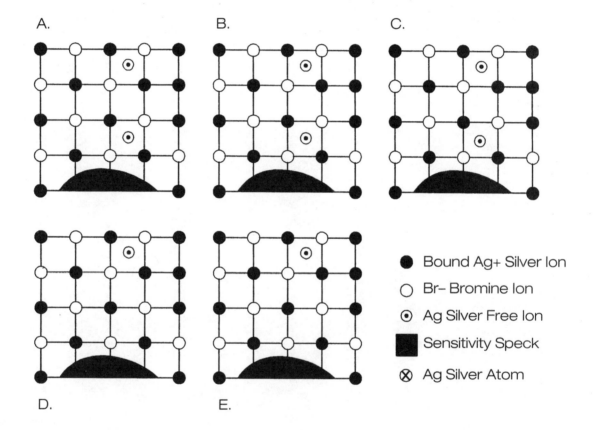

A.   B.   C.

D.   E.

- ● Bound Ag+ Silver Ion
- ○ Br– Bromine Ion
- ⊙ Ag Silver Free Ion
- ■ Sensitivity Speck
- ⊗ Ag Silver Atom

1. On Figure A draw an incident photon striking a bromide ion. Also draw an electron ejected from the resulting interaction.

2. On Figure B draw the ejected electron where it migrates after the interaction.

3. On Figure C draw the movement of a free silver ion to the sensitivity speck.

4. On Figure D show the final step in the process of latent image formation.

5. On Figure E show an accumulation large enough to result in a black metallic silver deposit when development occurs.

6.   What type of interaction must occur between the incident photon and the bromide ion in Figure A?

7.   Where does the ejected electron migrate in Figure B?

8.   Why is the free silver ion attracted to the sensitivity speck in Figure C?

9.   What occurs in Figure D?

LABORATORY 19-2   RADIOGRAPHIC DUPLICATION AND LIGHTENING TECHNIQUES

PURPOSE

Duplicate a diagnostic quality radiograph accurately and correct a radiograph that is too dark by overexposing duplication film.

MATERIALS

1. Diagnostic quality radiograph
2. Radiograph that is approximately 2–3X too dark
3. Radiographic duplication unit
4. Duplication film
5. Automatic film processor
6. Densitometer

EXPOSURE FACTORS

Suggested Factors

1–2 seconds

PROCEDURES

DUPLICATION

1. Use the procedure detailed in Figure 19–8 in the textbook to duplicate the diagnostic quality radiograph.

LIGHTENING

1. Use 15 seconds more than the exposure time that produced the duplicate film to duplicate the dark radiograph.

2. Continue to duplicate the dark radiograph at 15 second exposure increases until a diagnostic quality duplicate has been produced.

RESULTS

DUPLICATION

1. Select an average density area on the diagnostic quality radiograph (i.e., soft tissue between the sacrum and body of L5 on an abdomen, lung field between 3rd and 4th ribs in the apices of a chest, etc.). Use a densitometer to measure this area on both original and duplicated radiograph. Record the OD levels for both. If necessary, repeat the duplication procedure until these levels are within OD 0.30 of one another. (Remember that increased time will decrease density on duplication film and vice versa.)

2. Record the OD level for a light and dark area of both films.

LIGHTENING

1. Record on each film the exposure time used.

2. Record the OD levels for the same average density area on each of the films. Record these OD readings on the D log E graph below.

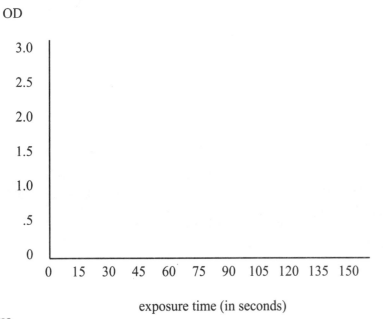

OD

exposure time (in seconds)

ANALYSIS

DUPLICATION

1. How much difference (in OD #) did you record between the original and duplicated film for the light area? for the average area? for the dark area?

2. Are the two images identical in contrast? If not, why?

LIGHTENING

1. According to the data on your D log E curve, what is the relationship between time and density when using duplicating film?

2. Construct a duplicating exposure time technique chart for lightening images that are too dark.

LABORATORY 19–3   SUBTRACTION TECHNIQUES

PURPOSE

Produce a subtraction image.

MATERIALS

1. Angiogram preliminary scout film
2. Angiogram contrast medium image from same series as scout
3. Radiographic subtraction unit
4. Subtraction mask film
5. Subtraction print film
6. Automatic film processor
7. Densitometer

SUGGESTED EXPOSURE FACTORS

See procedures.

PROCEDURES

1. Place the preliminary scout radiograph on the glass plate of the subtraction unit.

2. Under safelight conditions, place an unexposed subtraction mask film emulsion down (notch in LL corner) over the scout radiograph. Close and latch the lid to achieve good film-to-film contact and expose the film in the subtraction mode for 5 seconds.

3. Remove both films from the glass plate. Process the subtraction mask film.

4. Evaluate the mask film for sufficient density. Sufficient density is an average density similar to the original image. Repeat steps 1 and 2 until sufficient density is achieved. (Remember that a darker image is achieved by increasing exposure time.)

5. Place the mask film emulsion up on the glass plate of the subtraction unit and turn on the view light.

6. Place the contrast medium radiograph over the mask film and align the two images until the maximum subtraction of densities is achieved. Most densities should appear as a uniform density from the combination of the two opposite emulsions with only the contrast medium remaining in high contrast. Secure the alignment of the two images with masking tape.

7. Under safelight conditions, place an unexposed subtraction print film emulsion down (notch in LL corner) over the two aligned films. Close and latch the lid to achieve good film-to-film contact and expose the film in the subtraction mode for 10 seconds.

8. Remove all three films from the glass plate. Process the subtraction print film.

RESULTS

1. Evaluate the subtraction print film for sufficient density. Sufficient density is evaluated for the contrast medium injected vasculature only. The surrounding structures should be extremely light gray or nearly transparent. Repeat steps 5–8 until sufficient density is achieved. (Remember that exposure time must be increased with subtraction print film to produce a darker image.) Subtraction print film produces black vasculature. White vasculature can be produced by substituting duplication film for subtraction print film during the final exposure.

ANALYSIS

1. Compare the original contrast medium film with the subtraction film. Describe the structures that are visible on the original contrast medium film that do not appear on the subtraction film. Describe the structures that are visible on the subtraction film that do not appear on the original contrast medium film.

2. List specific projections from various radiographic procedures where subtraction techniques may provide additional diagnostic information.

LABORATORY 20-1   RADIOGRAPHIC PROCESSING AND CHEMISTRY

PURPOSE

Demonstrate the effects of time and temperature on radiographic density and contrast.

MATERIALS

1. Automatic film processor
2. Sensitometer
3. Photographic thermometer
4. 8" x 10" radiographic film
5. Densitometer

PROCEDURES

1. In the darkroom with the white lights off, write the number 1 on a sheet of 8" x 10" radiographic film using a lead pencil. Expose the film with a sensitometer.

2. Turn on a processor that has not been running for some time (it is necessary that developer temperature be less than optimal). Immediately process film #1. Record the developer temperature by using the photographic thermometer immersed in the developer tank.

3. Wait for developer temperature to reach normal operating level. Repeat step 1, but mark the film #2.

4. Develop film #2. Measure and record the temperature of the developer by using a photographic thermometer immersed in the developer tank.

5. Repeat step 1, but mark the film #3.

6. Feed film #3 into the processor. Exactly 10 seconds after the trailing end of the film has entered the processor, turn the processor off for exactly one minute. At the end of the 60 seconds, turn the processor back on.

7. Using a densitometer, measure the ODs of the steps for film #2. Locate the step number closest to an OD of 1.2 and identify this step as the speed step. Record the OD measured at the speed step along with the OD of the second step above the speed step in the results section. **NOTE:** The step # identified as the speed step for film #2 must also be used for films #1 and #3.

8. Use a densitometer to measure the ODs of the assigned speed step and second step above the speed step on films #1 and #3 and record the measurements in the results section.

RESULTS

	Film # 1	Film # 2	Film # 3
OD of speed step # (Density)	_____	_____	_____
OD of second step above speed step	_____	_____	_____
Difference between the two steps (Contrast)	_____	_____	_____

ANALYSIS

1. Assuming that the radiographic density (speed step) and contrast (difference between the two OD measurements) of film #2 represent optimal image quality, summarize the effects that development temperature and time have on radiographic density and contrast.

2. Modern automatic film processors complete the development stage of the film processing sequence in approximately 20 seconds, while manual film processing requires 3 to 5 minutes for the development stage to be completed. Explain why these times are so different.

3. List the stages of the automatic processing sequence and explain the function of each stage.

4. List the components of developer solution and give the function of each.

5. List the components of fixer solution and give the function of each.

PURPOSE

Identify and critically examine the function of the listed automatic processor parts or systems, processor malfunctions, and recommend appropriate corrective action.

MATERIALS

1. Automatic film processor

PROCEDURES

The instructor will identify and explain the principle of each of the following:

1. feed tray
2. entrance rollers
3. drive motor system
4. recirculation system
5. transport racks
    developer, fixer, and wash
    turnarounds
6. crossover networks
    labels, alignment, and
    guide shoes
7. dryer tubes
8. immersion time

9. water requirements
    consumption and filters
10. temperature
    adjustments
    heat exchanger
    dryer temperature
11. replenishment
    rate adjustments
    line filters
    oxidation covers
12. standby unit
13. silver recovery connection

RESULTS

1. Using the following diagram of a modern automatic radiographic film processor, fill in the blanks with the appropriate components.

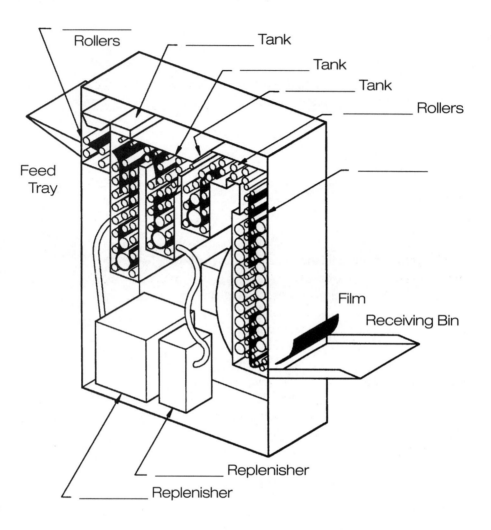

_____ Rollers

_____ Tank

_____ Tank

_____ Tank

_____ Rollers

_____

Feed
Tray

Film

Receiving Bin

_____ Replenisher

_____ Replenisher

ANALYSIS

1. What are the functions of the replenishment and recirculation systems? How are they similar? different?

2. Discuss the significance of water temperature as it affects developer temperature. In most processors (non-cold water models) what are the common limits of water temperature as related to the desired developer temperature?

3. What is the function of the heat exchanger? Where is one located?

4. Calculate the water saved by using a standby unit. Assume an automatic processor operates 40 hours per week for 52 weeks per year and uses 2–1/2 gallons of water per minute. How many gallons of water would be used during the 1 year period? If you added a standby unit, it would reduce the volume of water used during the non-operational times of the processor. Assume that during the 40 hour processor work week, the processor is in the standby mode for 5 hours per day. Water use during the 5 hours standby mode is 1 gallon per minute. How many gallons of water are saved over a full year? Be sure to consider the fully operational time and the time spent in stand-by.

5. What advantages are there to having a standby unit? What are the disadvantages?

6. Explain how you could identify the diameter of a scratched roller from the processed radiograph.

7. How can you determine whether scratches on a radiograph are caused by the guide shoes of a crossover or by the turnaround?

8. In your clinic you have undertaken a recent contract that will greatly increase the number of 8" x 10" radiographs processed. What consideration should be given to changing replenishment rates per 14" x 17" film if the total number of films per day remains unchanged? Why?

9. List and describe three different types of silver recovery units that are used on automatic radiographic film processors.

LABORATORY 21-1   RADIOGRAPHIC FILM CHARACTERISTICS

PURPOSE

Evaluate film contrast and speed.

MATERIALS

1. Automatic film processor
2. 3 different types of orthochromatic film
3. Sensitometer
4. Densitometer
5. Graph paper

PROCEDURES

1. Ask your lab instructor for three different radiographic films. In the darkroom mark one film with the letter A and the others with the letters B and C. These identification letters should be used any time you are describing a particular film.

2. Expose the 3 films in a sensitometer. Expose one edge of the film then turn it over and expose the opposite edge of the film. This will expose both sides of the emulsion.

3. Make sure the developer temperature is at the optimal temperature, then process all the films at one time.

4. Use a densitometer to read and record the densities of each of the sensitometric steps on both emulsion sides of each of the three films. In addition obtain the base plus fog level for each film by measuring a cleared area on the film. Average the densities obtained on each side for every step. Use the averaged step density reading.

5. Use graph paper to construct a sensitometric curve for each film. Graph all 3 films on the same graph with each in a different color.

6. Analyze the sensitometric curves constructed for each film. Record the data necessary to calculate the average gradient (contrast) and relative speed for each film on the film characteristics data form. Remember that net density is the density delivered to the film by the exposure itself (the density above the base plus fog).

7. Use the recorded data to calculate the average gradient (contrast) for each film from a net density of 0.25 to 2.5. Show the calculations and record the solutions on the data form.

RESULTS

FILM CHARACTERISTICS DATA FORM

	FILM A	FILM B	FILM C
BASE + FOG			
LOG RELATIVE EXPOSURE @ NET DENSITY 0.25			
LOG RELATIVE EXPOSURE @ NET DENSITY 2.5			
LOG RELATIVE EXPOSURE @ NET DENSITY 1.0			
FILM CONTRAST			

CALCULATIONS

ANALYSIS

1. What is base plus fog? What impact does it have on film characteristics?

2. Which film exhibited the highest film contrast? the least? How did you calculate the contrast values?

3. What can be said relative to the exposure latitude of the three films? the film latitude?

4. Which film exhibited the highest film speed? the least?

5. Assume that it took 20 mAs to achieve a net density of 1.0 on film A. How much mAs would be required to achieve a net density of 1.0 on Film B? Film C?

6. What is the relationship between film speed and contrast? Does your data support this?

7. What is the relationship between film latitude and contrast? Does your data support this?

PURPOSE

Demonstrate the color and intensity of light emitted from intensifying screens and evaluate the effect of film and screen spectral emission on film/screen combination speed.

MATERIALS

1. Energized radiographic unit
2. Automatic film processor
3. Calcium tungstate cassettes
4. Green light emitting rare earth cassettes (including detail)
5. Blue and green sensitive film
6. Step wedge (penetrometer)
7. Densitometer

SUGGESTED EXPOSURE FACTORS

100 RS, 100 mA, 0.125 sec, 75 kVp, 40" SID, non grid

PROCEDURE A

1. Obtain the following unloaded cassettes: one slow speed (50 RS) calcium tungstate, one high speed (200 RS) calcium tungstate, one slow speed (100 RS) green emitting rare earth, and one regular speed (400 RS) green emitting rare earth.

2. Open the cassettes and arrange them on the table so a corner of each of the four open cassettes is common to the others. Note the relative speed of each of the different cassettes.

3. Using a 40" SID, center the x-ray tube to the point where all four corners meet and open the collimator as wide as possible so as to include as much of each of the four cassettes as possible.

4. Turn off the lights in the exposure room and while observing the radiographic table through the viewing window of the control booth, make an exposure using 75 kVp, 100 mA, for 4 sec.

PROCEDURE B

1. Obtain one slow or detail green light emitting rare earth cassette. Load the cassettes with blue sensitive radiographic film and identify the cassettes appropriately.

2. Place the cassette on the radiographic table and center the step wedge on the cassette so that it is perpendicular to the anode cathode axis of the x-ray tube. Center and collimate the beam to the step wedge. Expose using the suggested exposure factors and process the film.

3. Using the same cassette, load it with orthochromatic (green sensitive) radiographic film and identify the cassettes appropriately.

4. Repeat procedure step 2.

5. Use a densitometer to measure the optical densities (OD) of the steps on each of the radiographs and record them on the appropriate data form.

6. Use the densitometer to measure the base + fog level of each radiograph. Subtract the base + fog value from the optical density readings for each film and record the results (net OD) on the data form.

RESULTS

SPECTRAL EMISSION AND SENSITIVITY DATA FORM

Screen Emission	Green			
Film Sensitivity	Blue		Green	
Step Number	OD	Net OD	OD	Net OD
1				
2				
3				
4				
5				
6				
7				
8				
9				
10				

ANALYSIS

1. Describe the intensity (brightness) of the light given off by the four cassettes. Does there appear to be any correlation between the light intensity and the speed of the screens exposed? Explain.

2. Describe the color(s) of the light emitted by the screens. Does there appear to be any correlation between the color of light emitted and the screen phosphor type? Explain.

3. Is there a speed difference between the green and blue film exposed in the green cassette? Explain.

4. Do you feel that the speed difference is significant? Why?

5. Do you feel that basically the same results would occur if you exposed a blue and green light sensitive film in a blue light emitting cassette? Explain.

LABORATORY 22-2   CASSETTE AND FILM HANDLING

PURPOSE

Illustrate the correct procedure for loading and unloading cassettes.
Demonstrate artifacts that result from common film mishandling situations.

MATERIALS

1. Automatic film processor
2. Cassette with scrap and fresh film to match size
3. Empty film box to match size of film
4. Cigarette lighter
5. Hand lotion

PROCEDURES

1. In a lighted environment place a cassette on a flat surface with the back (latch side) facing up. Practice releasing the cassette latches, opening the cassette so that the back side falls away from you. Close the cassette gently making sure the latches are fully engaged by pressing on the back. Next repeat the sequence with your eyes closed. Follow this exercise a number of times until you feel comfortable in accomplishing the task.

2. Obtain a sheet of scrap film and an empty film box of the appropriate size for the cassette being used. Place the scrap film in the box and set the box on the floor next to a table. Place the cassette on the table.

3. Practice loading and unloading the cassette with the film utilizing the following procedures:

    Loading Procedure—Open the cassette and grasp the film in the box with your thumb and first finger. Lift the film from the box. Once the film has cleared the box, grasp the opposite edge of the film with the thumb and first finger of your other hand. Position the film over the recessed portion of the open cassette and gently lower the film into the cassette. Make sure the film is seated in the recessed area of the cassette, then close the cassette.

    Unloading Procedure—Open the loaded cassette, laying the back flat on the table. With one hand lift the front side of the cassette toward the rear or latch side, allowing the film to fall free from the cassette. Grasp the edge of the film with the thumb and first finger of your other hand and lift, lowering the cassette front back to the table. Grasp the opposite edge of the film with the thumb and first finger of your free hand. The film should be transported with opposite edges held between the thumb and first finger of both hands or with the film held vertically with the thumb and first finger of one hand.

4. Practice the loading and unloading sequence with your eyes closed until you are comfortable with the task.

5. Under darkroom conditions, lay a single sheet of fresh film on the darkroom bench. Pick up the film and grasp it between your thumb and the first two fingers of one hand. Make a conscious effort to squeeze and kink the film. Next drop the film on the dark room floor, slide it across the floor, and step on it.

6. Step away and while facing the bench, light the cigarette lighter and quickly extinguish it.

7. Apply some hand lotion to your fingers. Pick up the film and grasp one edge with your fingers. Wipe the lotion off your fingers and wet your hands. Pick up the film and grasp the other edge with your wet fingers, then process the film.

RESULTS

1. Review the processed film for the presence of artifacts.

ANALYSIS

1. Why is it best to lay the film in the cassette rather than to slide it in when loading?

2. Why is it best to permit the film to drop into your fingers rather than to pick it out when unloading?

3. Why is it best to grasp the film between the thumb and first finger rather than between the thumb and first two fingers when handling and transporting film?

4. Why is it best to transport film holding it vertically rather than horizontally when using one hand?

5. Why is it best to grasp the opposite sides of the film using both hands rather than grasping one edge with one hand?

6. What is a film artifact? Why are they of concern?

7. Describe the artifacts present on the film. Match each artifact with the mishandling that caused it.

8. Describe other artifacts that can occur.

LABORATORY 23-1   **EVALUATING RADIOGRAPHIC FILM/SCREEN COMBINATIONS**

PURPOSE

Determine appropriate film/screen combinations for various clinical situations, formulate basic technical factors, and approximate exposure for various film/screen combinations.

MATERIALS

1. Energized radiographic unit
2. Densitometer
3. Automatic film processor
4. Various different intensifying screens in cassettes
5. Various films compatible with the screens
6. Radiographic phantom (i.e., skull or knee)
7. Resolution test tool
8. Step wedge (penetrometer) with marker or dot on a middle step
9. Dosimeter (digital ion chamber recommended)

SUGGESTED EXPOSURE FACTORS

RS (see procedure), 15 mAs, 80 kVp, 40" SID, non grid
The mA station must not vary between exposures (100 mA recommended).

PROCEDURES

1. Expose a control film of the following items with a single exposure:

   > phantom in lateral position
   > resolution tool (under phantom)
   > aluminum step wedge (next to phantom)
   > dosimeter ion chamber

   The marked step of the step wedge must exhibit an optical density (OD) of 1.30 to 1.70. If necessary, adjust the exposure factors and repeat until the OD standard has been achieved. Time changes are recommended although kVp can be modified if necessary to achieve the OD range. Record the OD of the marked step and the dose reading in mR and then develop normally.

2. Repeat step 1 using at least one other film and one other set of intensifying screens until at least 4 different film/screen combinations have been produced.

RESULTS

1. Complete the data in the following table.

combination		mAs	OD	lp/mm	mR
film	screen				

ANALYSIS

1. Rank the film/screen combinations according to the mAs required to produce similar densities on the film. Why did you need to use different mAs for different film/screen combinations?

2. Rank the film/screen combinations according to approximate exposure dose that a patient would have received (use your mAs ratings). Describe any correlation between mAs and exposure.

3. Using the lp/mm rankings, describe any correlation between the mAs and the resolving power of the system. Describe any relationship between the resolution and exposure.

4. Recommend film/screen combinations for each of the following clinical situations when maximum resolution is required. Use good judgment on contrast, latitude, and exposure.

(a) portable chest radiography

(b) general emergency room radiography

(c) newborn intensive care unit abdominal radiography

(d) serial filming of cerebral angiography

(e) navicular wrist magnification radiography

5. Repeat step 4 with patient exposure as the primary requirement.

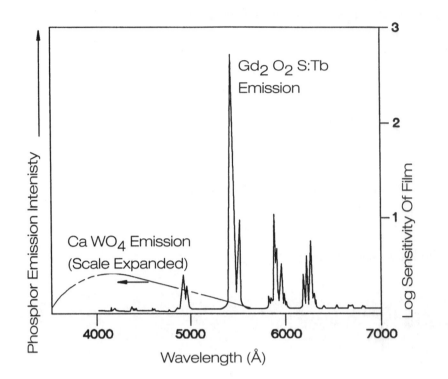

6. Draw in an approximate curve for blue sensitive film and another curve for green sensitive film on the graph above. Below what wavelength would both films produce an image? Above what wavelength would only the green sensitive film produce an image?

LABORATORY 24-1   EVALUATING ACCEPTANCE LIMITS

PURPOSE

Describe approximate diagnostic image quality acceptance limits.

MATERIALS

1. Energized radiographic unit
2. Abdomen or pelvis phantom
3. 14" x 17" cassette

SUGGESTED EXPOSURE FACTORS
(for 1st exposure)

RS 400, 2.5 mAs, 80 kVp, 40" SID, 8:1 grid

PROCEDURES

1. Produce a series of phantom images ranging from extremely light to completely dark by 2X mAs increments (i.e., use exposures of 2.5, 5, 10, 20, 40 mAs, etc. until the image of the phantom is completely dark).

RESULTS

1. Clearly number the images from lightest to darkest and arrange the entire series on view boxes in order of density.

2. Survey as many radiologists, administrative and supervising technologists, radiographers, and students as possible. Ask each professional to record only those images that could not be accepted for diagnosis. The goal is to determine which images could be submitted for diagnosis, not which is the best image.

3. Construct a histogram on the graph below by drawing vertical bars to indicate how many persons indicated they would submit each image for diagnosis.

4. Construct similar histograms for each group of professionals for whom results were obtained (i.e., radiologists, administrators, radiographers, students, etc.).

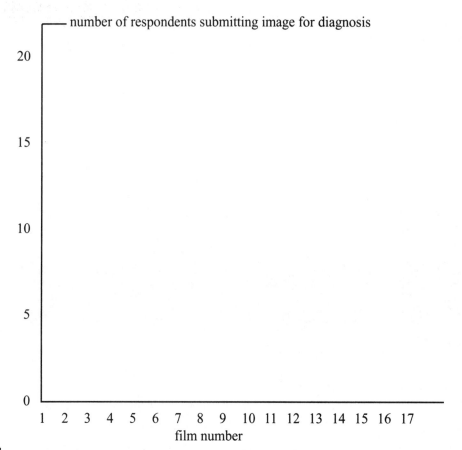

ANALYSIS

1. Compare the histograms for the different groups and discuss why the groups are similar or different.

2. Compare your personal opinion of the images to the results you obtained for each group. Explain possible reasons for all differences.

3. Give your opinion as to the total results of your study as compared to the general examples in Chapter 24 of the textbook.

LABORATORY 25-1   THE EFFECT OF mA AND TIME ON DENSITY

PURPOSE

Demonstrate the effect of mA and time on radiographic density.

MATERIALS

1. Energized radiographic unit
2. Automatic film processor
3. 10" x 12" radiographic cassettes and film
4. Wrist phantom
5. Step wedge
6. Densitometer

SUGGESTED EXPOSURE FACTORS

100 RS, see procedures for mA and sec, 60 kVp, 40" SID, non grid

PROCEDURES

mA

1. Place a 10" x 12" cassette crosswise on top of the radiographic table. Using lead masks divide the cassette into thirds in a crosswise fashion for three exposures on one film.

2. Center the wrist phantom and step wedge on the unmasked portion. Label the film A, center the CR, and collimate the beam to the unmasked portion of the film. Make an exposure at 60 kVp, 50 mA, 1/20 sec, and 40" SID.

3. Rearrange the masks to reveal the middle third of the cassette and repeat step 2. Adjust the mA to 100 and make an exposure.

4. Rearrange the masks to reveal the final third of the cassette and repeat step 2. Adjust the mA to 200 and make an exposure.

5. Process film A.

6. Using a densitometer, measure and record the OD of step 6 of the step wedge images.

Time (sec)

1. Place a 10" x 12" cassette crosswise on top of the radiographic table. Using lead masks divide the cassette into thirds in a crosswise fashion for three exposures on one film.

2. Center the wrist phantom and step wedge on the unmasked portion. Label the film B, center the CR, and collimate the beam to the unmasked portion of the film. Make an exposure at 60 kVp, 100 mA, 1/10 sec, and 40" SID.

3. Rearrange the masks to reveal the middle third of the cassette and repeat step 2. Adjust the exposure time to 1/20 sec, and make an exposure.

4. Rearrange the masks to reveal the final third of the cassette and repeat step 2. Adjust the exposure time to 1/40 sec, and make an exposure.

5. Process film B.

6. Using a densitometer, measure and record the OD of step 6 of the step wedge images.

mA and Time (sec)

1. Place a 10" x 12" cassette crosswise on top of the radiographic table. Using lead masks divide the cassette into thirds in a crosswise fashion for three exposures on one film.

2. Center the wrist phantom and step wedge on the unmasked portion. Label the film C, center the CR, and collimate the beam to the unmasked portion of the film. Make an exposure at 60 kVp, 5 mAs using 100 mA and 1/20 sec, and 40" SID.

3. Rearrange the masks to reveal the middle third of the cassette and repeat step 2. Select 5 mAs using 100 mA and 1/20 sec, and make an exposure.

4. Rearrange the masks to reveal the final third of the cassette and repeat step 2. Select 5 mAs using 200 mA and 1/40 sec, and make an exposure.

5. Process film C.

6. Using a densitometer, measure and record the OD of step 6 of the step wedge images.

RESULTS

OD step 6

	50 mA	100 mA	200 mA
Radiograph A	_____	_____	_____

OD step 6

	1/10 sec	1/20 sec	1/40 sec
Radiograph B	_____	_____	_____

OD step 6

	50 mA	100 mA	200 mA
	1/10 sec	1/20 sec	1/40 sec
Radiograph C	_____	_____	_____

ANALYSIS

1. As the milliamperage is increased, what effect is seen on the radiographic density of each of the three images?

2. What is the physical basis for the occurrence of these changes?

3. As the time of exposure is increased, what effect is seen on the radiographic density of each of the three images?

4. What is the physical basis for the occurrence of these changes?

5. What effect does the manipulation of milliamperes (mA) and exposure time (s) have on the radiographic density of each of the three images?

6. What is the physical basis for this occurrence?

LABORATORY 25-2   **THE EFFECT OF kVp ON DENSITY—THE 15% RULE**

PURPOSE

Demonstrate the effects of kilovoltage on density and the control of radiographic density by changing kVp and mAs utilizing the 15% rule.

MATERIALS

1. Energized radiographic unit
2. Automatic film processor
3. 14" x 17" cassette and film
4. Knee phantom
5. Step wedge
6. Densitometer

SUGGESTED EXPOSURE FACTORS

400 RS, see procedure for mA, sec, and kVp, 40" SID, non grid

PROCEDURES

A. kVp vs Density

1. Place a 14" x 17" cassette crosswise on top of the radiographic table. Using lead masks divide the cassette into thirds in a crosswise fashion for three exposures on one film.

2. Center the phantom knee and step wedge on the unmasked portion. Label the film A, center the CR, and collimate the beam to the unmasked portion of the film. Make an exposure at 75 kVp, 2 mAs and 40" SID.

3. Rearrange the masks to reveal the middle third of the cassette and repeat step 2. Change the kVp to 65 and expose the film.

4. Rearrange the masks to reveal the final third of the cassette and repeat step 2. Change the kVp to 86 and expose the film.

5. Process film A.

6. Using a densitometer, measure and record the OD of step 6 of the step wedge images.

B. 15% Rule for Density Control

1. Place a 14" x 17" cassette crosswise on top of the radiographic table. Using lead masks divide the cassette into thirds in a crosswise fashion for three exposures on one film.

2. Center the phantom knee and step wedge on the unmasked portion. Label the film B, center the CR, and collimate the beam to the unmasked portion of the film. Make an exposure at 75 kVp, 2 mAs and 40" SID.

3. Rearrange the masks to reveal the middle third of the cassette and repeat step 2. Decrease the kVp to 65 and, using the 15% rule, calculate the mAs to be used with the new kVp and expose the film.

4. Rearrange the masks to reveal the final third of the cassette and repeat step 2. Increase the kVp to 86 and, using the 15% rule, calculate the mAs to be used with the new kVp and expose the film.

5. Process film B.

6. Using a densitometer, measure and record the OD of step 6 of the step wedge images.

RESULTS

OD step 6

	75 kV	65 kV	86 kV
Radiograph A	_____	_____	_____
Radiograph B	_____	_____	_____

ANALYSIS

1. Discuss the density of the three images in procedure A using both visual and quantitative data.

2. Discuss the density of the three images in procedure B using both visual and quantitative data.

3. How do the visual and quantitative results in procedure B compare with the images obtained with similar kVp's in procedure A? Explain.

4. What is the theory behind the results in procedure B? Do your results support the theory? Explain.

5. What observations can you make about the contrast of the three images in procedure B? in procedure A?

LABORATORY 25-3   DETERMINING ADEQUATE PENETRATION

PURPOSE

Demonstrate the effects of x-ray penetration in regard to radiographic density and the visibility of the object radiographed.

MATERIALS

1. Energized radiographic unit
2. Automatic film processor
3. Abdomen phantom
4. 10" x 12" radiographic cassettes with film
5. Densitometer

SUGGESTED EXPOSURE FACTORS

400 RS, 200 mA, 0.2 sec, 70 kVp, 40" SID, 8:1 Bucky grid

PROCEDURES

1. Using a 10" x 12" cassette in the Bucky, position the phantom for an AP lumbar spine, with the CR centered to the iliac crest. Collimate to film size, expose, and process the film.

2. Repeat step 1 but reduce the kVp to 40 and increase the mAs to 600.

3. Repeat step 2 but increase the mAs to 1200.

RESULTS

1. Review the three films side by side, comparing the radiographic images for visibility of the spine and for radiographic density.

ANALYSIS

1. Has a satisfactory density been achieved and is the spine visible on radiograph #1? #2? #3?

2. Would a satisfactory density be achieved if the mAs is increased to 2000? 4000? Explain.

3. Can sufficient density and visibility of structures occur in the absence of proper penetration? Explain.

LABORATORY 25–4

THE EFFECT OF DISTANCE ON DENSITY—
THE DENSITY MAINTENANCE FORMULA

PURPOSE

Demonstrate the effect of SID on radiographic density and the use of the density maintenance formula to control radiographic density.

MATERIALS

1. Energized radiographic unit
2. Automatic film processor
3. 14" x 17" radiographic cassettes and film
4. Knee phantom
5. Step wedge (penetrometer)
6. Densitometer

SUGGESTED EXPOSURE FACTORS

400 RS, see procedure for mA, sec, and kVp, 40" SID, non grid

PROCEDURES

Distance and Density

1. Place a 14" x 17" cassette crosswise on top of the radiographic table. Using lead masks divide the cassette into thirds in a crosswise fashion for three exposures on one film.

2. Center the knee phantom and step wedge on the unmasked portion. Label the film A, center the CR, and collimate the beam to the unmasked portion of the film. Select 75 kVp, 2 mAs, and 40" SID, and expose the film.

3. Rearrange the masks to reveal the middle third of the cassette and repeat step 2. Adjust the SID to 60" and expose the film.

4. Rearrange the masks to reveal the final third of the cassette and repeat step 2. Adjust the SID to 20", expose the film, and process it.

5. Use a densitometer to measure and record the OD of step 6 of the step wedge.

Density Maintenance Formula

1. Place a 14" x 17" cassette crosswise on top of the radiographic table. Using lead masks divide the cassette into thirds in a crosswise fashion for three exposures on one film.

2. Center the knee phantom and step wedge on unmasked portion. Label the film B, center the CR, and collimate the beam to the unmasked portion of the film. Select 75 kVp, 2 mAs, and 40" SID, and expose the film.

3. Rearrange the masks to reveal the middle third of the cassette and repeat step 2. Increase the SID to 60" and, using the density maintenance formula, calculate the mAs to be used with the new distance to maintain the density and expose the film.

4. Rearrange the masks to reveal the final third of the cassette and repeat step 2. Decrease the SID to 20" and, using the density maintenance formula, calculate the mAs to be used with the new distance, expose, and process the film.

5. Use a densitometer to measure and record the OD of step 6 of the step wedge.

RESULTS

OD step 6

	40"	60"	20"
Radiograph A	___	___	___
Radiograph B	___	___	___

ANALYSIS

1. As the SID is increased what effect is seen in the density of each of the three images on radiograph A?

2. What is the physical basis for the changes seen on radiograph A?

3. What effect does the manipulation of mAs have on density (radiograph B)?

4. What is the physical basis for the results demonstrated on radiograph B?

5. Briefly describe the practical importance of the mAs/distance relationships as seen on radiograph B.

LABORATORY 25–5   THE EFFECT OF FILM/SCREEN COMBINATIONS ON DENSITY

PURPOSE

Demonstrate the effect of different radiographic film/screen combinations on radiographic density.

MATERIALS

1. Energized radiographic unit
2. Automatic film processor
3. Various speed cassettes
4. Knee phantom
5. Densitometer
6. Step wedge (penetrometer)

SUGGESTED EXPOSURE FACTORS

See procedure for RS, 100 mA, 0.05 sec, 70 kVp, 40" SID, non grid

PROCEDURES

1. Produce an image of the knee phantom and step wedge with each of the following film/screen combinations. Use the same exposure factors for each with the CR centered and perpendicular to the knee, the step wedge parallel to the knee, and the beam collimated to the cassette size.

    a. Detail (100 RS)   c. Regular (400 RS)
    b. Medium (250 RS)   d. Fast (800 RS)

2. Use a densitometer to record the OD of the middle step (step 6) of each of the four step wedge images.

RESULTS

	OD step 6
Detail	_____
Medium	_____
Regular	_____
Fast	_____

ANALYSIS

1. What inferences can be made from the differences in the densities on each of the radiographs?

2. Did the densities appear to follow a uniform progression? Explain.

3. What physical factors dictate the speed (sensitivity) of an intensifying screen?

4. How do screen manufacturers vary the speed of intensifying screens during their construction?

5. What is the purpose of having such a wide variety of screen speeds available?

LABORATORY 25-6   **THE EFFECT OF SUBJECT DENSITY AND CONTRAST ON DENSITY**

PURPOSE

Demonstrate the effect of different subject densities and contrast on radiographic density.

MATERIALS

1. Energized radiographic unit
2. Automatic film processor
3. 8" x 10" radiographic cassettes with film
4. Shallow container (about 3"–4" deep)
5. Ice cubes
6. 35 mm film canister
7. Super ball 1" diameter
8. Barium solution

SUGGESTED EXPOSURE FACTORS

100 RS, see procedure for mAs and kVp, 40" SID, non grid

PROCEDURES

NOTE: The films produced for this laboratory are also used for laboratory 26-3, The Effect of Subject Density and Contrast on Contrast.

Subject Density and Radiographic Density

1. Fill the container with enough ice cubes to form a single layer. Add water to equal the height of the ice cubes.

2. Mask a cassette in half, center the container to the unmasked portion, collimate, label film #1 and expose at 45 kVp, 1.25 mAs, and 40" SID.

3. Add water to increase the depth to 2" in the container. Use the other half of the cassette to repeat steps 2 and 3 and process the film.

Subject Contrast and Radiographic Density

1. Place a super ball in an empty 35 mm film canister. Fill the canister with water and replace the cap. Fill the shallow container with water to a depth of 3" and add the film canister.

2. Mask a cassette in quarters, center the container to an unmasked portion, collimate, label film #2, and expose at 70 kVp, 8 mAs, and 40" SID.

3. Remove the water from the film canister and replace the super ball and cap. Place the film canister in the shallow container, change the mask, and repeat step 2.

4. Fill the film canister with a liquid barium suspension, replace the super ball and the cap to the film canister. Place the film canister in the shallow container. Change the mask and repeat step 2.

5. Remove the barium from the film canister, rinse well with water, replace the super ball in the empty film canister, and replace the cap. Change the mask and center the film canister directly to an unmasked quarter of the cassette (do not place the film canister in the shallow container). Center, collimate, and expose using 70 kVp, 1 mAs, and 40" SID.

6. Process the film.

RESULTS

1. Review the images on both radiographs for radiographic density.

ANALYSIS

1. What caused the different densities seen in radiograph #1?

2. Why are fewer densities seen in the second image on radiograph #1?

3. Which image demonstrates the greatest number of densities on radiograph #2? Why?

4. Which image demonstrates the least number of densities on radiograph #2? Why?

5. Assuming the super ball is a solid tumor, which of the first three images demonstrates its density the best? Why?

LABORATORY 26-1   THE EFFECT OF kVp ON CONTRAST

PURPOSE

Demonstrate the effects of kVp on image contrast.

MATERIALS

1. Energized radiographic unit
2. Automatic film processor
3. 10" x 12" cassette with film
4. Step wedge
5. Skull phantom
6. Densitometer

SUGGESTED EXPOSURE FACTORS

400 RS, 100 mA, 0.33 sec, 60 kVp, 40" SID, 8:1 Bucky grid

PROCEDURES

1. Use a 10" x 12" cassette to produce a lateral skull with a step wedge adjacent to it.

2. Use a densitometer to record the OD of steps 4, 5, and 6 of the step wedge. If the OD of step 5 is not 1.2 ± 0.2, adjust the mAs and re-expose.

3. Repeat steps 1 and 2 using 80 kVp, 15 mAs and 40"SID.

4. Repeat steps 1 and 2 using 96 kVp, 7.5 mAs and 40"SID.

RESULTS

1. Record the OD of steps 4, 5, and 6 below.

2. Calculate the radiographic contrast of each image by subtracting the OD of step 6 from the OD of step 4.

kVp	Step Wedge Optical Density			Contrast
	Step 4	Step 5	Step 6	Step 4–Step 6
60	_____	_____	_____	_____
80	_____	_____	_____	_____
96	_____	_____	_____	_____

ANALYSIS

1. Compare the overall radiographic density of each radiograph individually and then compare the overall densities between the radiographs. Describe your observations. Does your data support your findings? Explain.

2. Describe the observed differences in the contrast between the three radiographs. Explain the reason for the results. Does your data support your observations? Explain.

3. Why do you think it would be advantageous to be able to change the contrast of a radiograph?

4. Define radiographic contrast.

5. Explain the difference between long scale and short scale contrast.

LABORATORY 26-2   THE EFFECT OF FILM/SCREEN COMBINATIONS ON CONTRAST

PURPOSE

Demonstrate the effect that different screen speeds have on radiographic contrast.

MATERIALS

1. Energized radiographic unit
2. Automatic film processor
3. Various speed cassettes of same phosphor type with same film type
4. Step wedge (penetrometer)
5. Densitometer

SUGGESTED EXPOSURE FACTORS

See procedure.

PROCEDURES

1. Center a cassette on the table top. Position the step wedge on the cassette so it is perpendicular to the anode-cathode axis of the x-ray tube.

2. Make the exposures as suggested below or as otherwise given by your instructor. Make sure the film is permanently identified as to the speed of the screens. Repeat this procedure for each of the remaining film/screen systems and process all films.

Screen Type	Relative Speed	Step Wedge Exposure Factors
Fine	100	75 kVp, 25 mA, 1/15 sec
Medium	250	75 kVp, 25 mA, 1/30 sec
Regular	400	75 kVp, 25 mA, 1/40 sec
Fast	800	75 kVp, 25 mA, 1/60 sec

3. Using a densitometer, measure the OD (optical density) of steps 4, 5, and 6 on the penetrometer for all the radiographs. Record the OD readings. The OD of step 5 should be 1.2 ± 0.2 for all 4 images. If not, adjust the mAs and re-expose.

RESULTS

1. Record the optical density measurements of steps 4, 5, and 6 below.

2. Calculate the radiographic contrast of each image by subtracting the OD of step 6 from the OD of step 4.

Screen	RS	Step Wedge Optical Density			Contrast
		Step 4	Step 5	Step 6	Step 4–Step 6
Fine	100	_____	_____	_____	_____
Medium	250	_____	_____	_____	_____
Regular	400	_____	_____	_____	_____
Fast	800	_____	_____	_____	_____

ANALYSIS

1. Were the differences in contrast of the four images significant? Explain.

2. Based on your data, what conclusions can you draw about the effect of screen speed on radiographic contrast?

3. Would you expect to see a difference in radiographic contrast between screens of the same speed and phosphor type but matched with different film? Explain.

4. Would you expect to see a difference in contrast between screens of the same speed but of different phosphor types? Explain.

LABORATORY 26–3   THE EFFECT OF SUBJECT DENSITY AND CONTRAST ON CONTRAST

PURPOSE

Demonstrate the effect of different subject densities and contrast on radiographic contrast.

MATERIALS

1.   Energized radiographic unit
2.   Automatic film processor
3.   8" x 10" radiographic cassettes with film
4.   Shallow container (about 3"–4" deep)
5.   Ice cubes
6.   35 mm film canister
7.   Super ball 1" diameter size
8.   Barium solution

SUGGESTED EXPOSURE FACTORS

100 RS, see procedure for mAs and kVp, 40" SID, non grid

PROCEDURES

Use the films produced for laboratory 25-6, The Effect of Subject Density and Contrast on Density. If laboratory 25-6 was not done previously, use the procedures section from that laboratory to produce the films for this laboratory.

RESULTS

1.   Review the images on both radiographs for radiographic contrast.

ANALYSIS

1.   What caused the different contrast ranges seen in radiograph #1?

2.   Why was the contrast reduced in the second image on radiograph #1?

3. Which image demonstrates the greatest contrast on radiograph #2? Why?

4. Which image demonstrates the least contrast on radiograph #2? Why?

5. Assuming the super ball is a solid tumor, which of the first three images demonstrates its contrast the best? Why?

LABORATORY 26-4   THE EFFECT OF EXPOSURE LATITUDE ON CONTRAST

PURPOSE

Demonstrate how exposure latitude affects radiographic contrast.

MATERIALS

1. Energized radiographic unit
2. Automatic film processor
3. 10" x 12" radiographic cassettes with film
4. Hand phantom

SUGGESTED EXPOSURE FACTORS

100 RS, see procedure for mAs and kVp, 40" SID, non grid

PROCEDURES

1. Mask a cassette in half crosswise and center it to the top of the radiographic table. Center the hand phantom to the unmasked portion of cassette, label it exposure #1, collimate to the film size, and expose using 45 kVp and 20 mAs.

2. Repeat step #1, labeling it exposure #2, expose using 55 kVp and 20 mAs, and process the film.

3. Repeat steps #1 and #2. Label the first half exposure #3 and expose using 73 kVp and 5 mAs. Label the second half exposure #4 and expose using 83 kVp and 5 mAs. Process the film.

4. Repeat steps #1 and #2. Label the first half exposure #5 and expose using 96 kVp and 1 mAs. Label the second half exposure #6 and expose using 106 kVp and 1 mAs. Process the film.

RESULTS

1. Review radiographs with respect to radiographic density and contrast.

ANALYSIS

1. Is the background density similar on all three radiographs?

2.   Which radiograph demonstrates the lowest contrast? What is the reason for this?

3.   Which radiograph demonstrates the highest contrast? What is the reason for this?

4.   Which radiograph demonstrates the greatest difference between the contrast of the two images? Explain.

5.   Which radiograph demonstrates the least difference between the contrast of the two images? Explain.

6.   Summarize the effect that kVp has on exposure latitude using the laboratory results to support your statements.

7.   Explain the practical clinical application that is supported by the results of this laboratory activity.

LABORATORY 26–5

THE EFFECT OF GRIDS ON CONTRAST

PURPOSE

Demonstrate the effectiveness of radiographic grids in the improvement of contrast.

MATERIALS

1. Energized radiographic unit
2. Automatic film processor
3. Low and high ratio radiographic grids
4. Abdomen phantom
5. 14" x 17" radiographic cassettes with film
6. Step wedge (penetrometer)
7. Densitometer

SUGGESTED EXPOSURE FACTORS

400 RS, 200 mA, 0.03 sec, 75 kVp, 40" SID, non grid

PROCEDURES

1. Center the abdomen phantom to the cassette on the table top. Place the step wedge beside the phantom on the cassette. Direct the central ray perpendicular and collimate to the edges of the cassette.

2. Using the suggested exposure factors expose the film, process, and label it #1.

3. Use a densitometer to measure the OD of steps 4, 5, and 6 on the penetrometer and record the readings. The OD of step 5 should be 1.2 ± 0.2. If not adjust the mAs and re-expose.

4. Repeat the procedure using a low ratio grid. Expose the film using the appropriate grid conversion factor, process, and label it #2.

5. Repeat the procedure using a high ratio grid. Expose the film using the appropriate grid conversion factor, process, and label it #3.

6. Calculate the radiographic contrast of each image by subtracting the OD of step 6 from the OD of step 4.

RESULTS

1. Review the three radiographs in terms of their radiographic density and contrast.

	Step Wedge Optical Density			Contrast
	Step 4	Step 5	Step 6	Step 4–Step 6
Radiograph #1	_____	_____	_____	_____
Radiograph #2	_____	_____	_____	_____
Radiograph #3	_____	_____	_____	_____

ANALYSIS

1. Compare the radiographic densities and contrast of radiographs 1, 2 and 3. Which radiograph(s) more closely approximate(s) a quality image? Why?

2. Where are the differences in radiographic contrast of the three images significant? Explain.

3. Based on your data, what conclusions can you draw about the effect of grids and grid ratio on radiographic contrast?

4. What factors or influences have contributed to the decrease or increase of image quality in each of the radiographs?

5. Why is a radiographic grid important?

LABORATORY 27-1   THE EFFECT OF DISTANCE ON RECORDED DETAIL

PURPOSE

Demonstrate the effects of object film distance and source image receptor distance on recorded detail.

MATERIALS

1. Energized radiographic unit
2. 8" x 10" cassettes and film
3. Dry bone parts
4. Radiolucent sponges
5. Lead masks
6. Resolution test pattern
7. Film processor

SUGGESTED EXPOSURE FACTORS

100 RS, 100 mA, 0.017 sec, 55 kVp, 40" SID, non grid

PROCEDURES

1. Mask a cassette in half and place the test pattern and a dry bone on a 2" radiolucent sponge on the unmasked portion of cassette. Center the bone and test pattern to the unmasked half, label it exposure #1, collimate to the edges of the unmasked area, and expose using 55 kVp, 3 mAs, and 40" SID.

2. Readjust the mask to the other half of the cassette, center the bone and test pattern on top of an 8" sponge on the unmasked portion of the cassette, label it exposure #2, collimate to the unmasked area, expose using the same technical factors, and process the film.

3. Place a cassette on the floor, mask it in half and place the test pattern and dry bone on an 8" radiolucent sponge on the unmasked portion of the cassette. Center the bone and test pattern to the unmasked half, label it exposure #3, collimate to the edges of the unmasked area, and expose using 55 kVp and 60" SID with the mAs adjusted according to the density maintenance formula (as derived from the inverse square law) to maintain the same density as the first film.

4. Readjust the mask to the other half of the cassette, repeat step 3 using 80" SID, label it exposure #4, and process the film.

RESULTS

1. Review all four radiographic images. Compare the recorded detail of both the bone and the test pattern images. Carefully determine the image of the smallest group where the line pairs can be distinctly defined (separated) and record the lines/mm of the group below.

<u>Smallest group resolved (lines/mm)</u>

40" SID/2" OID _____

40" SID/8" OID _____

60" SID/8" OID _____

80" SID/8" OID _____

ANALYSIS

1. Is there an obvious loss of recorded detail between the first two exposures of the bone? Which image demonstrates the best recorded detail?

2. On exposures #1 and #2, is the recorded detail loss as great in the test pattern as with the bone? Explain the reasons for the difference, if any. Indicate the greatest number of lines/mm demonstrated on each exposure.

3. Describe the recorded detail of exposures #2 and #3. What is the greatest number of lines/mm that you can clearly see? What causes this difference? Explain.

4. Describe the effect of SID as it relates to image definition. Of what practical value is this knowledge to the radiographer?

LABORATORY 27–2   THE EFFECT OF FOCAL SPOT SIZE ON RECORDED DETAIL

PURPOSE

Demonstrate the effect of focal spot size on recorded detail.

MATERIALS

1. Energized radiographic unit
2. Automatic film processor
3. 8" x 10" cassette and film
4. Dry bones
5. Resolution test pattern
6. Radiolucent sponge

SUGGESTED EXPOSURE FACTORS

100 RS, 100 mA, 0.017 sec, 55 kVp, 40" SID, non grid

PROCEDURES

1. Ascertain that the exposure factors to be used can be obtained with both a small and large focal spot. If not, locate a radiographic unit capable of satisfying this requirement.

2. Mask the cassette in half, center a dry bone and the test pattern on a 2" thick radiolucent sponge to the unmasked side, label exposure #1, collimate, and expose using the small focal spot.

3. Repeat step 2 on the other half of the cassette, label exposure #2, expose using the large focal spot, and process the film.

RESULTS

1. Review both images. Compare the recorded detail of both the bone and the test pattern images. Carefully determine the image of the smallest group where the line pairs can be distinctly defined and record the lp/mm below.

<u>Smallest group resolved (lp/mm)</u>

Small Focal Spot   _____

Large Focal Spot   _____

ANALYSIS

1. Is there an obvious loss of recorded detail between the two images of the bone? Which image demonstrates the best detail?

2. Is there an obvious loss of recorded detail between the two resolution test patterns? Indicate the greatest number of lp/mm that you can see clearly defined in each of the images.

3. Is this loss as appreciable as that demonstrated in the images of the bones? Explain the reasons for your conclusion.

LABORATORY 27-3   THE EFFECT OF FILM/SCREEN COMBINATIONS ON RECORDED DETAIL

PURPOSE

Demonstrate the effect of different radiographic film/screen combinations on recorded detail.

MATERIALS

1. Energized radiographic unit
2. Automatic film processor
3. Various speed cassettes with film
4. Hand phantom
5. Resolution test pattern
6. Radiolucent sponge

SUGGESTED EXPOSURE FACTORS

See procedure.

PROCEDURES

1. Place the line pair test tool on a 2" radiolucent sponge, position it next to the phantom hand, expose a film with each of the three different intensifying screens listed below using a 40" SID and the suggested exposure factors, and process the films.

100 RS (fine)	54 kVp, 25 mA, 3/20 sec
400 RS (regular)	54 kVp, 25 mA, 1/20 sec
800 RS (fast)	54 kVp, 25 mA, 1/40 sec

RESULTS

1. Review all three radiographs. Compare the recorded detail of both the hand and the test pattern images. Carefully determine the image of the smallest group where the line pairs can be distinctly defined (separated) and record the lines/mm of the group below.

<u>Smallest group resolved (lines/mm)</u>

100 RS   _____

400 RS   _____

800 RS   _____

ANALYSIS

1. Is the difference in recorded detail displayed on the three radiographs more noticeable with the hand images or the test pattern images. Why?

2. Which radiograph exhibits the best recorded detail? Support your choice by describing the images.

3. Which radiograph demonstrates the poorest recorded detail? Support your choice by describing the images.

4. List the factors associated with intensifying screens that have an impact on recorded detail and use these factors to explain the results you obtained.

5. What clinical trade-off is apparent when selecting a screen that produces better recorded detail?

LABORATORY 27–4   THE EFFECT OF MOTION ON RECORDED DETAIL

PURPOSE

Demonstrate the effect of object motion on recorded detail.

MATERIALS

1. Energized radiographic unit
2. Automatic film processor
3. Non-screen film holder with film
4. Hand phantom
5. String

SUGGESTED EXPOSURE FACTORS

Direct exposure, 100 mA, 3.0 sec, 62 kVp, 40" SID, non grid

PROCEDURES

1. Mask a non-screen film holder in half, center the hand phantom to the unmasked area, direct a perpendicular CR to the center of the hand, collimate to the unmasked section, and expose.

2. Remask to the other half and repeat step 1 with the hand in motion. Motion can be achieved by tying to the phantom a piece of string of sufficient length to reach the control booth and gently pulling the phantom during the exposure. (It is best to practice several times before making the exposure.) Then process the film.

RESULTS

1. Review both radiographic images. Consider the recorded detail of each image.

ANALYSIS

1. Is there a difference between the recorded detail of the two images? If a difference is noted, describe it.

2. Why does motion reduce recorded detail?

3. List the two types of patient motion associated with radiographic imaging. Give two methods that could be used to control each type.

● **LABORATORY 28-1**   **THE EFFECT OF DISTANCE ON SIZE DISTORTION**

PURPOSE

Demonstrate the effect of OID and SID on size distortion.

MATERIALS

1. Energized radiographic unit
2. Automatic film processor
3. 10" x 12" cassette with film
4. Small dry bone (vertebra preferred)
5. Metric ruler

SUGGESTED EXPOSURE FACTORS

100 RS, 100 mA, 0.017 sec, 55 kVp, 40" SID, non grid

PROCEDURES

OID PROCEDURE
1. Mask a cassette in quarters, center a dry bone on a 2" thick radiolucent sponge to the unmasked area, label exposure #1, collimate, and expose.

2. Repeat step 1 on an unmasked area using another sponge to increase the OID to 4", label exposure #2, and expose.

3. Repeat step 1 on an unmasked area using another sponge to increase the OID to 8", label exposure #3, and expose.

4. Repeat step 1 on an unmasked area using another sponge to increase the OID to 12", label exposure #4, expose, and process the film.

SID PROCEDURE

1. Mask a cassette in quarters, center a dry bone on a 2" thick radiolucent sponge to the unmasked area, change the SID to 20", use the density maintenance formula (as derived from the inverse square law) to adjust the exposure factors, label exposure #1, collimate, and expose.

2. Repeat step 1 on an unmasked area using 30" SID, use the density maintenance formula to adjust the exposure factors, label exposure #2, and expose.

3. Repeat step 1 on an unmasked area using 40" SID, use the density maintenance formula to adjust the exposure factors, label exposure #2, and expose.

4. Repeat step 1 on an unmasked area using 60" SID (this distance is best obtained by placing the cassette on the floor), use the density maintenance formula to adjust the exposure factors, label exposure #2, and expose.

RESULTS

1. Accurately record the length of the dry bone and the images from the various exposures.

2. Calculate and record the magnification factor and percentage of magnification for each image.

OID DATA FORM

DRY BONE (OBJECT) LENGTH (OL) = _____mm   SID = _____

OID	BONE IMAGE LENGTH (IL) (mm)	magnification factor (m) $\dfrac{SID}{SID-OID}$	% Magnification (% M) $\dfrac{IL-OL}{OL} \times 100$
2"			
4"			
8"			
12"			

SID DATA FORM

DRY BONE (OBJECT) LENGTH (OL) = _____mm   OID = _____

OID	mAs	BONE IMAGE LENGTH (IL) (mm)	magnification factor (m) $\dfrac{SID}{SID-OID}$	% Magnification (%M) $\dfrac{IL-OL}{OL} \times 100$
20"				
30"				
40"				
60"				

ANALYSIS

1. What happens to the recorded size of the image as the OID increases?

2. At what point does the loss of image detail become unacceptable? Explain.

3. What happens to the recorded size of the image as the SID increases?

4. At what point does the loss of image detail become unacceptable? Explain.

5. Describe the role of SID in producing size distortion and indicate how you would use this information to advantage to produce an image with minimal size distortion.

6. Compare the results of the two procedures. Which factor produces the greatest influence on size distortion? Support your answer.

7. Do the magnification factor and percentages compare favorably? Explain.

8. What effect does size distortion have on recorded detail?

LABORATORY 28-2   THE EFFECT OF ALIGNMENT AND ANGULATION ON SHAPE DISTORTION

PURPOSE

Demonstrate the effect of part/film alignment, CR/part/film alignment and CR direction on shape distortion.

MATERIALS

1. Energized radiographic unit
2. Automatic film processor
3. 10" x 12" cassette with film
4. Dry bone
5. Metric ruler

SUGGESTED EXPOSURE FACTORS

100 RS, 100 mA, 0.017 sec, 55 kVp, 40" SID, non grid

PROCEDURES

Part/Film Alignment

1. Position a 10" x 12" cassette lengthwise on the table top so the ID blocker is down, mask the cassette in thirds lengthwise, tape the dry bone on a 4" sponge so that the long axis of the bone is parallel to the tube axis, center the bone to an unmasked area, direct the CR to the center of the bone with a 40" SID, label exposure #1, and expose.

2. Repeat step 1 on an unexposed area, center the bone to the area, direct the CR to the center of the bone with a 40" SID, raise the right (cathode) end of the sponge so the bone forms a 30° angle with the film plane, label exposure #2, and expose.

3. Repeat step 1 on an unexposed area, center the bone to the area, direct the CR to the center of the bone with a 40" SID, raise the left (anode) end of the sponge so the bone forms a 30° angle with the film plane, label exposure #3, expose, and process the film.

CR/Part/Film Alignment

1. Position a 10" x 12" cassette lengthwise on the table top so the ID blocker is down, mask the cassette in thirds lengthwise, tape the dry bone on a 4" sponge so that the long axis of the bone is parallel to the tube axis, center the bone to an unmasked area, direct the CR to the center of the bone with a 40" SID, label exposure #4, and expose.

2. Repeat step 1 on an unmasked area, center the bone to the area, direct the CR to the left (toward the anode) along the longitudinal axis of the bone until it is 6" off-center, open the collimator to include the entire bone, label exposure #5, and expose.

3. Repeat step 1 on an unmasked area, center the bone to the area, direct the CR to the right (toward the cathode) along the longitudinal axis of the bone until it is 6" off-center, open the collimator to include the entire bone, label exposure #6, expose, and process the film.

<u>CR Direction</u>

1. Position a 10" x 12" cassette lengthwise on the table top so the ID blocker is down, mask the cassette in thirds lengthwise, tape the dry bone on a 4" sponge so that the long axis of the bone is parallel to the tube axis, center the bone to an unmasked area, direct the CR to the center of the bone with a 40" SID, label exposure #7, and expose.

2. Repeat step 1 on an unmasked area, center the bone to the area, direct the CR to the left (toward the anode) along the longitudinal axis of the bone until it is 6" off-center, angle back 25° to the original centering point, reduce the SID to 40", label exposure #8, and expose.

3. Repeat step 2 on an unmasked area, direct the CR to the right (toward the cathode) along the longitudinal axis of the bone until it is 6" off-center, angle back 25° to the original centering point, reduce the SID to 40", label exposure #9, expose, and process the film.

RESULTS

1. Accurately measure the length of the dry bone and the images of the bone on the film and record them in mm.

Dry Bone Length _____mm   Bone Image Length (mm)

Part/Film Alignment	Image 1	Image 2	Image 3
	_____	_____	_____
CR/Part/Film Alignment	Image 4	Image 5	Image 6
	_____	_____	_____
CR Direction	Image 7	Image 8	Image 9
	_____	_____	_____

ANALYSIS

<u>Part/Film Alignment</u>

1. Compare the differences in anatomical appearance between the recorded images in which portions are elongated/foreshortened. Compare image 1–2, 1–3, 2–3.

2. Can shape distortion caused by improper part/film relationship also contribute to size distortion? Explain.

3. To minimize shape distortion, indicate the most ideal relationship between the structures of interest and the film plane.

CR/Part/Film Alignment

4. Compare the differences in anatomical appearance between the recorded images in which portions are elongated/foreshortened. Compare image 4–5, 4–6, 5–6.

5. Can shape distortion caused by improper CR/part/film alignment also contribute to size distortion? Explain.

6. Describe the significance of off-centering of the CR on the visualization of joint spaces or nondisplaced fractures.

CR Direction

7. Compare the differences in anatomical appearance between the recorded images in which portions are elongated/foreshortened. Compare image 7–8, 7–9, 8–9

8. Can shape distortion caused by improper CR direction through the part also contribute to size distortion? Explain.

9. Would it be more appropriate to direct the CR perpendicular to the film or to the structure of interest? Explain your answer and provide some practical examples that support your position.

10. Compare the shape distortion produced in the three different scenarios. Of the three causes of shape distortion identified, which produces the most obvious misrepresentation of the structure? Support your answer with examples.

11. Name three examinations/projections in which shape distortion is used to advantage and describe how this is accomplished.

LABORATORY 29-1

FILM CRITIQUE: ASSESSING DENSITY, CONTRAST, RECORDED DETAIL, AND DISTORTION

PURPOSE

Critique films effectively.

MATERIALS

1. A repeated radiograph

PROCEDURES

1. Use the procedures described in Chapter 29 of the textbook to critique the repeated radiograph using the following form.

FILM CRITIQUE FORM

I. CLASSIFY THE RADIOGRAPHIC IMAGE AS:
☐ **WITHIN ACCEPTANCE LIMITS**

☐ Optimal diagnostic information (critique is complete)

(all checkmarks below this line require completion of section II and III)

☐ Suboptimal diagnostic information

☐ **OUTSIDE ACCEPTANCE LIMITS**

II. DETERMINE THE CAUSE OF THE PROBLEM AS:
☐ **A: Technical Factors**

☐ Photographic problem with visibility of detail

☐ Density

☐ mAs_____

☐ Influencing factor (specify) _____

☐ Contrast

☐ kVp _____

☐ Influencing factor (specify) _____

☐ Geometric problem with detail

☐ Recorded detail

☐ Geometry (specify) _____

☐ Film/Screen combination (specify) _____

☐ Motion

☐ Distortion

☐ Size (Magnification) (specify) _____

☐ Shape (Part/Film/Tube Alignment) (specify) _____

☐ **B: Procedural Factors**

☐ Patient Positioning

☐ Tube Alignment _____

☐ Part Alignment _____

☐ Film Alignment _____

☐ Patient Preparation (specify) _____

☐ **C: Equipment Malfunction**

☐ Processing Equipment (specify) _____

☐ Radiographic/Fluoroscopic Equipment (specify) _____

III. RECOMMENDED CORRECTIVE ACTION For each cause specified above:

_____
_____
_____
_____

LABORATORY 30-1 PROCESSOR SENSITOMETRIC MONITORING CHARTS

PURPOSE

Monitor an automatic film processor sensitometrically.

MATERIALS

1. Automatic film processor
2. Sensitometer
3. Densitometer
4. Radiographic control film
5. Photographic thermometer

PROCEDURES

1. A quantity (box) of radiographic film that is normally used in the processor being monitored should be set aside to be used as control film, use this film when making the sensitometric control strips.

2. Using a sheet of film from the control box, expose the film in the sensitometer. Follow the sensitometer's instruction manual for the correct procedure.

3. Process the sensitometric film. If the monitoring activity is going to be over a period of time, then the test film should be processed in a like fashion each time (i.e., film orientation, feed tray position, etc.).

4. Measure the developer temperature using a photographic thermometer each time a control film is processed. Record the temperature reading in the appropriate section of the processor monitoring record.

5. Use the densitometer to measure and record the step numbers and their optical densities on the sensitometric control strip for the following monitoring parameters:

Contrast Index

The OD of the step closest to but not less than 2.20 OD minus the OD of the step closest to but not greater than 0.45 OD.

Speed Index

Step closest to 1.20 OD.

Base + Fog Index

Unexposed portion of test film or 1st step.

6. These procedures will be used to measure these parameters, assuming that the processor is currently operating normally. The parameters measured above will be considered the normal value for this activity. Record these measurements (step numbers and densities) in the appropriate section of the processor monitoring record.

7. Monitor a film processor over a period of 2–4 weeks. The processor should be tested at least once a day at a time during its active use, using freshly sensitized sensitometric control strips. Record the developer temperature and the OD of each of the parameters on the processor monitoring record each time a sensitometric control strip is processed.

   Acceptance Criteria

   Each parameter should test within control limits for the processor to be considered operating normally and consistently. The control limits are:

Contrast Index:	plus or minus 0.10 OD.
Speed Index:	plus or minus 0.10 OD.
Base + Fog Index:	plus or minus 0.05 OD.
Developer Temp:	plus or minus 1° F or 0.5° C

RESULTS

See the next page.

ANALYSIS

1. If this activity required you to monitor a processor over a period of time, did any of the parameters fall outside of the control limits? What was the cause? How was the situation corrected?

2. Why is it recommended that freshly sensitized sensitometric control strips be used rather than pre-sensitizing a quantity of strips and using them throughout the monitoring procedure?

3. What effect would you predict for the speed, contrast, and base + fog indexes if the following occurred?

   a. Five hundred 14" x 17" films are run through the processor instead of 500 intermixed sized films.

b. The incoming water supply to the processor was 95° F when it should be 90° F.

c. A cracked safelight filter was found.

4. Discuss the importance of processor maintenance and its impact on processor quality control.

MONTH _____ YEAR _____
PROCESSOR MODEL NO. _____
LOCATION _____
RECORDED BY _____

PROCESSOR
MONITORING
RECORD

DAY

1 3 5 7 9 11 13 15 17 19 21 23 25 27 29 31

SPEED STEP NO. _____

+0.20 _____
+0.15 _____
+0.10 _____
+0.05 _____
D
-0.05 _____
-0.10 _____
-0.15 _____
-0.20 _____

CONTRAST
STEP _____ -STEP _____

+0.20 _____
+0.15 _____
+0.10 _____
+0.05 _____
D
-0.05 _____
-0.10 _____
-0.15 _____
-0.20 _____

GROSS FOG STEP _____

+0.10 _____
+0.05 _____
D
-0.05 _____
-0.10 _____

DEVELOPER STANDARD TEMP._____ °

+10° _____
+ 5° _____
°
- 5° _____
-10° _____

LABORATORY 30–2   ESTIMATING FOCAL SPOT SIZE

PURPOSE

Evaluate focal spot size using a star x-ray test pattern.

MATERIALS

1. Energized radiographic unit
2. Automatic film processor
3. 1.5 or 2 degree star x-ray test pattern
4. 10" x 12" non-screen film holder with screen film
5. Small metric ruler

SUGGESTED EXPOSURE FACTORS

Screen film with direct exposure, 20 mAs, 75 kVp, 24" SID, non grid

PROCEDURES

1. Locate the tube identification plate attached to the x-ray tube housing of the unit being tested. Record the nominal (manufacturer's specification) focal spot sizes that are indicated on the plate for the x-ray tube. They often appear as simply single decimal numbers (for example, 0.6–2.0 to indicate 0.6 mm and 2.0 mm focal spots).

2. Activate the collimator localizer light of the x-ray tube being evaluated, place the star test pattern in contact with the face plate of the collimator so it is centered to the center, and rotate the star so one set of lead lines is parallel with the long axis of the tube and the other set is perpendicular. Tape the test pattern to the collimator face plate in this position.

3. Center the loaded film holder lengthwise on the radiographic table, mask it in half crosswise, adjust the CR perpendicular to the center of the unmasked area, label the anode and cathode sides of the film holder, use a 24" SID, collimate to the unmasked portion of the film holder, select the large focal spot, and expose.

4. Readjust the mask, repeat step 2 using the small focal spot, expose, and process the film. An OD of 1.2 –1.5 should be obtained if possible.

5. Determine the magnification (M) factor by dividing the diameter of the radiographic image of the star test pattern by the true diameter of the star test pattern.

6. Determine the point at which failure of resolution occurs. By viewing the image starting at the outer margin of the star pattern, move inward to the first area of blurring and mark this point. Mark the point where failure of resolution occurs on all four sides. Measure the distance in millimeters between the two marks along the anode cathode axis (D_1) to determine the width of the focal spot. Measure the distance in millimeters between the two marks perpendicular to the anode cathode axis (D_2) to determine the length of the focal spot.

7. Calculate the equivalent focal spot size (F_{mm}) according to the following formula:

$$F_{mm} = \frac{N}{57.3} \times \frac{D}{(M-1)}$$

where:

N = the angle of the star pattern used for the evaluation i.e., 1.5 or 2

D = distance between failure of resolution marks in mm

M = magnification factor

F_{mm} = equivalent focal spot size in mm

RESULTS

	Small Focal Spot	Large Focal Spot
Nominal Size	_____	_____
Equivalent Size	_____	_____

ANALYSIS

1. What are the measured equivalent sizes of the large and small focal spots?

2. How do these figures compare to the nominal (manufacturer specified) focal spot size for the tube evaluated? If they are larger, do they meet the acceptable tolerance limits specified by NEMA (see textbook Chapter 6)? Explain.

3. Describe another method that can be used to evaluate focal spot size.

4. Describe the differences between effective, equivalent, and actual focal spot size.

LABORATORY 30–3   EVALUATING COLLIMATOR, CENTRAL RAY, AND BUCKY TRAY ALIGNMENT

PURPOSE

Evaluate the alignment of the light field and central ray to the x-ray beam and Bucky tray as well as the accuracy of the automatic collimation system.

MATERIALS

1. Energized radiographic unit equipped with PBL
2. Automatic film processor
3. Various size radiographic cassettes with film
4. One sheet of scrap film for each cassette size
5. Four paper clips
6. Collimator alignment template or 9 pennies
7. X-ray beam perpendicularity test tool

SUGGESTED EXPOSURE FACTORS

400 RS, 25 mA, 0.05 sec, 55 kVp, 40" SID, non grid

PROCEDURES

Light field x-ray beam alignment and perpendicularity

1. Center the alignment template on the cassette and place it on the table top.

2. Center the light field to the cross centering mark on the template using 40" SID.

3. Switch the PBL to manual mode and adjust the collimator light field to the field marks on the template.

4. If the light field is centered to the template, and one or more of the edges of the light field are not on the corresponding field marks, place straightened paper clips on the edges of the light field to mark the location.

5. Place the perpendicularity test tool on the template, making sure it is exactly centered to the template and to the center of the light field.

6. Place ID markers on the table top in the quadrant of the light field that represents the right shoulder of a supine patient for orientation purposes in the event misalignment is noted and expose the film.

7. Open the collimator to cover the entire film, expose a second time using half the mAs (this will be a double exposure), and process the film.

8. Evaluate the film for x-ray beam to light field alignment.

1. Federal guidelines for certified equipment allow ± 2% of the SID for x-ray beam to light field alignment. The edges of the radiation field should be within ± 1 cm of the template markers indicating the location of the light field edges.

2. The image of the BBs in the perpendicularity test tool should appear within 5 mm of one another.

Nine-penny test for beam alignment

1. Center a 10" x 12" cassette on the x-ray table top with its long dimension parallel to the long dimension of the table.

2. Center the light field to the center of the cassette at a 40" SID.

3. Manually collimate the x-ray beam to a 6" x 8" field size.

4. Position two pennies in the center of each margin of the light field so that one entire penny is inside the light field and one is outside the light field. Place the ninth penny in the quadrant of the light field that represents the right shoulder of a supine patient as an orientation marker.

5. Place lead markers well inside the light field on the cassette to identify the room number and date and expose the film at about 55 kVp and 1.25 mAs.

6. Open the collimator and adjust light field size to the cassette and expose the cassette again using 55 kVp and 0.5 mAs (this will be a double exposure), and process the film.

7. Evaluate the accuracy of the x-ray field.

Acceptance Limits

Federal guidelines for certified equipment allow ± 2% of the SID for the x-ray to light field alignment. For a 100 cm (40") SID, ± 2 cm (1 penny) is acceptable. The x-ray to light field should be well within this guideline. Alignment to ± 1 cm (± 0.5 penny) can reasonably be achieved.

Field size vs. cassette size for automatic collimation (PBL) systems

1. Set the x-ray tube at the usual target-to-film distance used for Bucky radiographs.

2. Set the PBL selector to the automatic mode.

3. Insert each size of cassette commonly used in the Bucky tray lengthwise and then transversely. Visually check that the changes in the light field size occur with the changes in cassette size and that the size of the light field is appropriate by comparing the light field size to the film size using scrap film sheets.

Acceptance Limits

Federal guidelines for certified equipment allow ± 3% of the SID for PBL misalignment; however, a ± 1 cm is reasonably achievable.

<u>X-ray field and Bucky alignment</u>

1. Set the x-ray tube to the transverse center position.

2. Place straightened paper clips on the x-ray table top along the cross hairs of the collimator light field.

3. Insert a 10" x 12" cassette lengthwise in the Bucky tray. Collimate the beam to an 8" x 10" size with the long dimension parallel to the x-ray table top.

4. Place ID markers on the table top in the quadrant of the light field that represents the right shoulder of a supine patient for orientation purposes in the event misalignment is noted and expose using about 50 kVp and 5 mAs.

5. Measure the distance from the center of the radiographic image as indicated by the crossed paper clips to the edges of the exposed portion of the radiograph and to the edges of the film.

<u>Acceptance Limits</u>

The exposed portion of the radiograph should be centered to the film within ±1 cm in both length and width. The center indicated by the images of the crossed paper clips should actually be centered to the exposed portion of the radiograph to within ± 1 cm.

RESULTS

1. Evaluate all the test films against the acceptance criteria.

ANALYSIS

1. Was the radiation light field alignment within acceptable limits? Explain. Discuss the clinical implications of a misaligned radiation beam and light field.

2. Was the radiation beam centering and perpendicularity within acceptable limits? Explain. Discuss the clinical implications of misalignment of the center of the beam and a beam that is not perpendicular.

3. Was the PBL test within acceptable limits? If not, explain the unacceptable elements. Discuss the clinical implications of an improperly operating PBL device.

4. Was the Bucky tray beam center alignment within acceptable limits? Explain. Discuss the clinical implications

of an improperly aligned Bucky tray.

5.   List at least 4 causes of centering and radiation to light field misalignment.

LABORATORY 30–4   EVALUATING DISTANCE, CENTERING, AND ANGULATOR ACCURACY

PURPOSE

Evaluate the accuracy of an SID indicator, centering detent, and angulation indicator.

MATERIALS

1. Energized radiographic unit
2. Automatic film processor
3. 8" x 10" cassette with film
4. Quarter or other coin
5. Ring stand
6. Scrap film
7. Small ruler
8. Skull angulator or protractor
9. Small bubble level

SUGGESTED EXPOSURE FACTORS

400 RS, 100 mA, 0.0083 sec, 60 kVp, 40" SID, 8:1 Bucky grid

PROCEDURES

SID Indicator Accuracy

1. Set up the ring stand on table top 20" above the Bucky tray and center it on the table. Cut a 4" x 4" section from a scrap film and place it on the ring support. Center a quarter on the film, use the tube's SID indicator to position the tube 40" above the Bucky tray, center the CR to the quarter and collimate appropriately. Place an 8" x 10" cassette in the Bucky tray and center it to the CR, expose, and process.

2. Use a metric ruler to determine the diameter of the quarter (object size). Measure the diameter of the image of the quarter on the test film (image size). Calculate the SID using the following equation:

$$SID = \frac{\text{image size} \times OID}{\text{image size} - \text{object size}}$$

Tube Centering Detent Accuracy

1. Place the x-ray tube at the center detent position and visually inspect the tube housing from the end and front of the table to make sure it is not angled (a bubble level can be used for more accuracy). Turn on the light localizer and note the position of the cross hairs on the table top. The longitudinal cross hair should be aligned to the midline of the table.

Angulation Indicator Accuracy

1. Position the tube head so that the angulation indicator reads 0 degrees. Place the bubble level on top of the tube housing and determine if the bubble indicates a level tube position. Angle the tube in both directions and watch the indicator to see if it is accurate. A protractor or skull angulator can be used to verify the correct angle.

RESULTS

SID Indicator Accuracy

Indicated SID   _____

Calculated SID   _____

Tube Centering Detent Accuracy

Distance between cross hair
and table center line   _____

Angulation Indicator Accuracy

Angulation indicator reading
  with tube head leveled   _____

ANALYSIS

1. What is the calculated SID?

2. The SID indicator should be within ± 2% of the calculated SID to be considered accurate. What is the percentage difference between the indicated SID and the calculated SID? Does the SID indicator pass the accuracy test?

3. Did the light localizer cross hair align with the midline of the table with the tube in the detent position? If not, by how much was it off?

4. Assume that the table did not have a center line. Describe a way that could be used to determine the accuracy of the detent mechanism.

5. Did the angulation indicator read 0 degrees with the tube head in a level position? If not, by how much was it off?

6. Describe at least one adverse effect that could result from each of the three parameters if they tested as being inaccurate.

LABORATORY 30–5   **EVALUATING KILOVOLTAGE ACCURACY**

PURPOSE

Evaluate the accuracy of kVp production.

MATERIALS

1. Energized radiographic unit
2. Automatic film processor
3. Digital kVp meter or kVp test cassette (with current calibration curve)
4. Densitometer (required with kVp test cassette)

SUGGESTED EXPOSURE FACTORS

See procedure.

PROCEDURES

Digital kVp Meter

1. The kVp settings evaluated should represent common kVp and mAs settings. Evaluate 60, 70, 80, 90, and 100 kVp at two different mA stations. If the generator is used for fluoroscopy, evaluate 120 instead of 60 kVp.

2. Set the meter for radiographic testing and for three-phase or single-phase depending on the type of generator. Most meters should be warmed up by an exposure of about 100 mAs and 100 kVp.

3. Position the meter on the table so the LCD readout is visible from the control booth, the detector is centered to the x-ray beam at 40" source to detector distance, and collimate to approximately 6" x 6".

4. Set the desired kVp, use 100 ms or longer for three-phase generators and 200 ms or longer for single-phase generators (shorter exposure times—(down to 50 ms)—can be used without significant loss of accuracy), and expose.

5. Record the results. If no indication of sufficient intensity for a measurement occurs, decrease the source to detector distance or increase the mA. Do not change the kVp or time.

6. Repeat steps 3 through 5 for the remaining test exposures.

KVP Test Cassette

1. Follow the manufacturer's directions for specific information such as film type to be used with the test cassette, recommended SID, recommended mAs, etc.

2. Load the test cassette and place it on the table top so the long axis of the cassette is parallel to the anode–cathode axis of the x-ray tube. Center and collimate the x-ray beam to the cassette using the manufacturer's recommendation or a 36" source-to-table top distance.

3. Set the generator to the mA station that will be used for all the kVp stations and identify the cassette with lead markers.

4. Mask the cassette in quarters and expose different areas of the cassette at 60, 80, 100, and 120 kVp. Adjust the time (not the mA) for each exposure so that an OD of 0.5 –1.5 is produced for each exposure and process the film.

   Approximate mAs techniques using Kodak TML film and 36" SID.

kVp	mAs	
	1 Phase	3 Phase
60	500	400
80	75	40
100	15	10
120	12	8

RESULTS

Digital kVp Meter

1. Record the kVp meter readings below.

Tested kVp	mA	Measured kVp
_____	_____	_____
_____	_____	_____
_____	_____	_____
_____	_____	_____
_____	_____	_____

2. The kVp on a properly calibrated generator should be maintained within ± 2 kVp. A variation of ± 5 kVp or more should be corrected by a service engineer.

kVp Test Cassette

1. Each kVp region on the film includes two columns of dots. Use a densitometer to measure the densities and record them on the data form. (The film must be repeated if the measured densities are not between OD 0.5–1.5.)

2. Locate the dot in the left (attenuation dot) column that most closely matches the densities in the right (reference dot) column.

3. Unless an exact match is found, interpolate between the steps to determine the appropriate match dot number, for example:

	Attenuation Density	Reference Density
Step 5	1.10	1.05
Step 6	1.03	1.05

$$\text{Match Step} = 5 + \frac{1.10 - 1.05}{1.10 - 1.03} = 5 + \frac{.05}{.07} = 5.7$$

4. If the reference dots are not uniform in the area of the density match, determine the average density for the reference dots close to where the match occurs and use this average density for matching purposes.

5. After the match step has been determined for each of the kVp regions (steps 2 and 3), refer to the cassette's calibration curves to determine the kVp. Every test cassette is matched to its own calibration curve. The serial number of the cassette must match the number on the calibration curves. There is a separate chart for each kVp region and there is a separate curve on each chart for single- and three-phase generators.

6. Record the results below.

Tested kVp	Match Dot	Measured kVp
————	————	————
————	————	————
————	————	————
————	————	————
————	————	————

7. The kVp on a properly calibrated generator should be maintained to within ± 2 kVp. A variation of ± 5 kVp or more should be corrected by a service engineer.

ANALYSIS

1. Were all the kVp settings tested within acceptable limits? If not, which ones were not and by how much?

2. Why is kVp considered such an important technical factor? Why must it be closely monitored?

3.   What is the reason for aligning the long axis of the test cassette with the long axis of the x-ray tube?

4.   Why do single- and three-phase generators require separate calibration curves to determine the kVp for this test?

5.   If a problem with kVp calibration is suspected, why would viewing the output waveform be helpful?

6.   What are two possible causes of kVp variations?

LABORATORY 30–6   **EVALUATING TIMER ACCURACY**

PURPOSE

Evaluate the accuracy of an exposure timer.

MATERIALS

1. Energized radiographic unit
2. Automatic film processor
3. Spinning top or motorized synchronous top
4. 8" x 10" radiographic cassettes with film
5. Timer protractor template or ordinary protractor

SUGGESTED EXPOSURE FACTORS

100 RS, 5 mAs, 75 kVp, 40" SID, non grid

PROCEDURES

Manual Spinning Top (for single-phase generators only)

1. Four exposures must be made using a constant mAs with varying mA and time. Typical values might be 0.2 sec @ 25 mA, 0.1 sec @ 50 mA, 0.05 sec @ 100 mA, and 0.03 sec @ 150 mA. Use mA stations that are commonly used with the generator.

2. Mask the cassette in quarters, collimate, center the top to the unmasked area, use 40" SID, mark it #1, start the top spinning, and make the first exposure.

3. Change the mask and repeat step 2 for the remaining areas, mark each appropriately, use different exposure factors for each, and process the film.

4. Count the dots for each image and record the results.

5. Determine the measured exposure time for each of the radiographs by dividing the number of dots by 120. Be sure to consider the type of rectification. Self-rectified generators produce 60 dots (pulses) per second while full-wave rectifiers produce 120 per second.

Acceptance Criteria

For tested time stations ≤ 0.1 sec, the image should display the exact pulse number. For tested time stations > 0.1 sec, the image should display the exact pulse number within ± 1 pulse.

Motorized Synchronous Top (for all types of generators)

1. The four exposures must be made using a constant mAs with varying mA and time. Typical values might be 0.2 sec @ 25 mA, 0.1 sec @ 50 mA, 0.05 sec @ 100 mA and 0.03 sec @ 150 mA. Use mA stations that are commonly used with the generator.

2. Plug the timing tool in, mask the cassette in half and collimate and center the top to the unmasked area, use 40" SID, mark it #1, start the top spinning, and make the first exposure.

3. Change the mask and repeat step 2 for the remaining areas, mark each appropriately, use different exposure factors for each, and process the film. Exposures #3 and 4 should be made with a second cassette.

4. Use the timer protractor template provided by the manufacturer to measure the angles of the darkened arcs, determine the time, and record it.

5. If the manufacturer's protractor template is not available, measure the angle of exposed arc using an ordinary protractor and use the following formula:

$$\frac{\text{Measured Angle}}{360° \times \text{RPS}} = \text{Exposure time}$$

Where RPS is the revolutions per second at which the motor operates. For example, a 36° arc with a 1 RPS synchronous motor would be calculated as:

$$\frac{36°}{360° \times 1} = 0.1 \text{ second}$$

Acceptance Criteria

For three-phase generators, exposure time error should be limited to ± 5% or ± 2 msec, whichever is larger.

RESULTS

Spinning Top

Time Station Tested	# Dots Displayed	Measured Exposure Time
_____	_____	_____
_____	_____	_____
_____	_____	_____
_____	_____	_____

Motorized Synchronous Top

Time Station Tested	Measured Angle	Measured Exposure Time
_____	_____	_____
_____	_____	_____
_____	_____	_____
_____	_____	_____

ANALYSIS

1. Were all the time stations evaluated within acceptable limits? If not, which ones were not and by how much?

2. What aspects of image quality are directly affected by exposure time?

3. A single-phase full-wave-rectified generator produces 3 dot images on the test radiograph. What exposure time would the results indicate?

4. A homemade motorized synchronous spin top operates at a speed of 78 rpm. A measured arc image of 8 degrees is produced when testing a particular three-phase generator. What exposure time is indicated by the result?

5. Why is a manual spin top contraindicated for determining exposure times for three-phase and high-frequency generators?

LABORATORY 30-7   EVALUATING EXPOSURE REPRODUCIBILITY, mA LINEARITY, AND mR/mAs

PURPOSE

Evaluate the reproducibility and linearity of a generator for commonly used exposure settings.

MATERIALS

1. Energized radiographic unit
2. Digital dosimeter (0–500 mR pen dosimeters can be substituted)

SUGGESTED EXPOSURE FACTORS

Choose a mAs that will produce dosimeter readings in the range of 200–500 mR at 80 kVp.

PROCEDURES

1. Turn on the digital dosimeter, select the dose mode, and follow the manufacturer's instructions for the unit's operation.

2. Place the dosimeter detector (ionization chamber) on the radiographic table, use a 40" source-to-detector distance, center and collimate the beam to the detector.

3. On the generator control panel, select 80 kVp, 100 mA, and an exposure time that will result in a dosimeter reading between 200 and 500 mR. Readjust the exposure time if necessary until the reading is within this range and record the values.

4. Randomly change the technical factor settings and then go back to the desired setting. Make three exposures and record the readings on the data form as X_1, X_2, and X_3 respectively.

5. Repeat steps 3 and 4, but use the next larger mA station (i.e., 200 mA).

6. Repeat steps 3 and 4, but use the next larger mA station (i.e., 300 mA).

7. Repeat steps 3 and 4, but use the next larger mA station (i.e., 400 mA).

8. In order to properly analyze the results of this test, certain simple calculations must be made and the results compared to the acceptance criteria.

   a. Calculate the average of the three exposure measurements made at each kVp, mA, and time combination and record on the data form.

   $$\text{Avg. } X = (X_1 + X_2 + X_3)/3$$

b. Calculate the average exposure per indicated mAs for each mA and time station tested as:

$$\text{Avg. mR/mAs} = \text{Avg. X}/(\text{mA} \times \text{s})$$

where Avg. X is the average value of the recorded exposures at each mA-time station combination and mA and s are the values of the stations selected. Record the calculated Avg. mR/mAs values on the data form.

c. For reproducibility calculate and record on the data form the ratios X_1/Avg. X, X_2/Avg. X, and X_3/Avg. X for each kVp, mA, and time combination.

Acceptance Criteria: For any specific combination of selected technique factors, the exposures shall provide reproducible exposure to 0.05 or less. Thus, at a given kVp, mA and time combination, the individual exposure measurements shall fall within ± 5% of the averages. This is indicated by X_n/Avg. X ratios between 0.95 and 1.05.

d. For linearity, use the calculated mR/mAs values to determine the linearity across all the mA stations selected at 80 kVp.

$$\text{Linearity} = [(\text{Avg. mR/mAs})_{max} - (\text{Avg. mR/mAs})_{min}]/[(\text{Avg. mR/mAs})_{max} + (\text{Avg. mR/mAs})_{min}]$$

where $(\text{Avg. mR/mAs})_{max}$ and $(\text{Avg. mR/mAs})_{min}$ are the maximum and minimum values of the calculated mR/mAs as recorded on the data form.

Acceptance Criteria: Essentially, linearity means that the ratio of exposure to total charge in mR/mAs is constant over the entire range of mAs values. The average mR/mAs obtained at any tube current settings (mA) shall not differ by more than 0.10. Linearity should be maintained to ±10% over the entire working range of the generator regardless of the number of mA stations at a fixed kVp.

9. Generator output is determined by taking the average of the four mR/mAs values. Average output produced by diagnostic x-ray equipment with a total filtration of 2.5 mm Al measured at 80 kVp with a 40" source-to-detector should be 5.0 mR/mAs for single phase and 8.0 mR/mAs for three phase.

Acceptance Criteria: The tested generator should agree with the average values to within ± 30 %, assuming other tests indicate proper performance, i.e., kVp, SID accuracy, HVL, etc.

RESULTS

1. Document the results of the test and calculations in the appropriate sections of the data form.

DATA FORM

mA									
TIME									
mAs									
X_1									
X_2									
X_3									
Avg. X									
X_1/Avg. X									
X_2/Avg. X									
X_3/Avg. X									
Avg.mR/mAs									

ANALYSIS

1. Did the test results meet the acceptance criteria for reproducibility of the mA, linearity across mA stations, and output? If not, indicate which tests failed and support your conclusions.

2. Briefly discuss the importance of the reproducibility and linearity tests.

3. What might be a cause for reproducibility being unacceptable? linearity?

4. Describe the benefits that can be derived from knowing the exposure output of the generators in a x-ray department. Why is exposure output expressed in mR/mAs?

LABORATORY 30–8   RADIOGRAPHIC CASSETTE QUALITY CONTROL

PURPOSE

Inspect and clean cassette screens and evaluate film/screen contact.

MATERIALS

1. Energized radiographic unit
2. Automatic film processor
3. Cassettes
4. Screen cleaner solution
5. Gauze sponge pads
6. Wire mesh test pattern
7. Adhesive tape

SUGGESTED EXPOSURE FACTORS

400 RS, small focus, 100 mA, 0.05 sec, 60 kVp, 40" SID, non grid

PROCEDURES

1. Visually inspect the cassette and screens. Give particular attention to the following:

    a. Loose, worn or broken hinges and catches.
    b. Locking straps or catches that are not holding securely.
    c. Warped, twisted, or cracked frames.
    d. Frayed or excessively worn or loose felt.
    e. Screens improperly installed in the cassette.
    f. Dust, dirt, scratches, chips, or stains on the screens.
    g. Deterioration of the screen's protective layer.

2. If the screens appear dirty or if they have not been cleaned recently, proceed as follows:

    a. Use screen cleaner solution or a mild soap and water solution to dampen a clean gauze sponge.

    b. Wipe one screen at a time with the gauze sponge in vertical lines, then repeat the process horizontally. After cleaning, wipe each screen with a dry gauze sponge.

    c. Leave cassettes open until the screens are <u>thoroughly dry.</u>

    d. Record the date on the appropriate label on the rear of the cassette, if none exists, fashion one out of tape and fasten it to the cassette with the necessary information recorded.

    e. If a screen cleaning log is kept, record the cassette number and date cleaned in the appropriate place.

3. Load a clean cassette with fresh film. Wait 5 minutes to ensure that any trapped air has escaped.

4. Place the cassette in the center of the radiographic table, center the tube to the cassette and collimate to the cassette size using a 40 inch SID.

5. Place the wire mesh test tool on top of the cassette. Expose the cassette using suggested exposure factors.

6. Process the film. A density of 1.2 to 1.5 should be obtained to make a proper evaluation. If necessary, repeat this step until the appropriate density is achieved.

RESULTS

1. Place the test radiograph on a radiographic illuminator in a dimly lit environment.

2. View the radiograph at a distance of six to nine feet.

3. Areas of poor film/screen contact will be demonstrated by areas of increased density or non-uniformity of density and a cloudy or hazy appearance.

4. Areas of poor contact that exist around the perimeter of the cassette may be considered acceptable provided they do not extend more than 1 inch into the film. Areas of poor contact in the center of the image are completely unacceptable.

5. For new cassettes the above criteria should be more rigid than for older cassettes.

ANALYSIS

1. Did the cassettes tested pass the film/screen contact test? If not, describe the appearance of the images.

2. What is the clinical importance of film/screen contact?

3. Give at least two reasons why it is essential to maintain screen cleanliness.

LABORATORY 30-9   **EVALUATING VIEW BOX UNIFORMITY**

PURPOSE

Evaluate the uniformity of radiographic view boxes (illuminators).

MATERIALS

1. Light meter
2. Test mask (14" x 17" cardboard with a hole cut in the center of each of four quadrants)
3. View boxes, at least two separate banks of multiple panels.

PROCEDURES

1. Clean any dirty view boxes, including inside, with a wet cloth.

2. Place the test mask on the view box to be evaluated. The mask is divided into 4 quadrants, each containing a hole for the light meter.

3. Position the light meter over the upper left quadrant and record the reading. Illumination (intensity) level can be measured as lux, foot-candle (fc), or eV, depending on the type of light meter being used.

4. Repeat step 3 for the other quadrants and record the readings.

5. Repeat procedures 1–4 for all other view box panels to be tested and record the appropriate data. Most view box panels are grouped together to form a bank. With this in mind it is sensible to test the variation of illumination level between the panels, which together form a bank. Since these banks of view boxes will be found in different areas around the radiology department it is also wise to test the variation in illumination levels between the separate banks of view boxes.

6. Record the room (ambient) light level for the viewing area.

7. Using the recorded test results, calculate and record the following:

    a. Determine the average illumination level for each view box panel.

    $$\text{Avg. } I_p = I_{q^1} + I_{q^2} + I_{q^3} + I_{q^4} / 4$$

    b. Determine the average illumination level for the entire bank of view box panels.

    $$\text{Avg. } I_B = \text{Avg. } I_{p^1} + \text{Avg. } I_{p^2} + \dots \text{Avg. } I_{p^n} / n$$

c. For each view box panel, determine the maximum variation in the illumination level between quadrants.

$$V_{IP} = (I_{q\,max} - I_{q\,min}) / (I_{q\,max} + I_{q\,min}) \times 100\%$$

d. Determine the maximum variation between the averages of the individual panels for a given bank of view boxes.

$$V_{IB} = (\text{Avg. } I_{p\,max} - \text{Avg. } I_{p\,min}) / (\text{Avg. } I_{p\,max} + \text{Avg. } I_{p\,min}) \times 100\%$$

e. Determine the maximum variation between the averages of different view box banks within a radiology department.

$$V_{IG} = (\text{Avg. } I_{B\,max} - \text{Avg. } I_{B\,min}) / (\text{Avg. } I_{B\,max} + \text{Avg. } I_{B\,min}) \times 100\%$$

RESULTS

VIEW BOX BANK _____

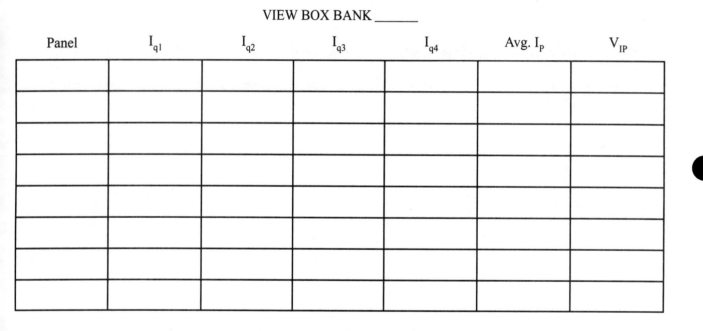

Panel	I_{q1}	I_{q2}	I_{q3}	I_{q4}	Avg. I_P	V_{IP}

Avg. I_B = _____ V_{IB} = _____   Ambient Light Level _____

<u>Acceptance Criteria</u>

View box illumination level: minimum of 500 fc or 13 eV at 100 ASA
Ambient room light level: maximum of 8 fc or 8 eV at 100 ASA

$V_{IP} \leq 10\%$ $V_{IB} \leq 15\%$ $V_{IG} \leq 20\%$

ANALYSIS

1. Did the ambient light level(s) for the view box(es) tested pass the acceptance criteria? If not, what was the % error?

2. What effect might an overly bright reading area have on viewing a radiograph?

3. Did all the view box panels tested pass the acceptance criteria for illumination level and uniformity? If not, which ones were not acceptable and what was the % error?

4. What effect might a dim view box have on viewing a radiograph?

5. What effect might the lack of illumination uniformity of a view box have on viewing a radiograph?

6. Did all the banks of view boxes tested pass the acceptance criteria for illumination uniformity between the panels? If not, which ones were not acceptable and what was the % error?

7. What effect might the lack of illumination uniformity between panels on a bank of view boxes have on viewing radiographs?

8. If separate banks of view boxes were tested, did they pass the acceptance criteria for illumination uniformity? If not, which ones were not acceptable and what was the % error?

9. What effect might the lack of illumination uniformity between banks of view boxes have on viewing radiographs?

10. Describe at least four possible causes for illumination problems associated with view boxes.

LABORATORY 30–10   **REPEAT FILM STUDIES**

PURPOSE

Analyze repeated radiographs in a radiology department.

MATERIALS

1. Radiographs repeated during a survey period
2. Repeat analysis worksheet

PROCEDURES

1. Establish a method to accurately determine the amount of film used (i.e., record films, multiply average films per exam by number of exams recorded, computerized film usage, etc.).

2. Set a start date and length for the survey period. Clean out all repeat film bins to begin the study. (A four-week survey period is recommended.)

3. At the end of the survey period collect all repeated radiographs and determine the total number of films used during this period.

4. Analyze the repeated radiographs to determine the reason that they were probably repeated using the categories listed on the repeat analysis worksheet.

RESULTS

1. Using the repeat analysis worksheet, record the number of repeated radiographs in each repeat category against the exam type they represent according to the exam categories listed on the next page.

ANALYSIS

1. Calculate the monthly repeat rate (%) based on the data collected for the survey period.

2. Calculate the repeat rate (%) of repeated films by repeat reason category.

3. Calculate the repeat rate (%) of repeated films by exam category.

4. List suggestions for corrective measures (actions) to minimize the repeat rates in the problem areas identified.

REPEAT ANALYSIS WORKSHEET

SURVEY PERIOD _____ to _____ LOCATION _____

REPEAT CATEGORY EXAM	POSITION	OVER-EXPOSED	UNDER-EXPOSED	MOTION	ARTI-FACTS	OTHER	TOTAL	%
CHEST								
RIBS								
SHOULDER								
HUMERUS								
ELBOW								
FOREARM								
WRIST								
HAND								
C-SPINE								
T-SPINE								
L-SPINE								
SKULL								
FACIAL								
SINUSES								
ABDOMEN								
PELVIS								
HIP								
FEMUR								
KNEE								
LOWER LEG								
ANKLE								
FOOT								
UGI								
LGI								
IVP								
OTHER								
TOTAL								
%								

LABORATORY 30-11   DARKROOM SAFELIGHT TEST

PURPOSE

Evaluate the safelight conditions and the sensitivity of exposed and unexposed radiographic film to a darkroom safelight.

MATERIALS

1.   Energized radiographic unit
2.   Film processor
3.   10" x 12" cassette and film
4.   10" x 12" piece of cardboard
5.   Densitometer

SUGGESTED EXPOSURE FACTORS

400 RS, 25 mA, 0.017 sec, 40 kVp, 40" SID, non grid

PROCEDURES

1.   Mask the cassette in half, center to the unmasked area, collimate, expose and process the film. Remove the film from the cassette in the darkroom in total darkness and lay it on the darkroom counter top.

2.   Place a piece of cardboard crosswise over entire film, leaving approximately one inch at the top. Place a small pencil mark on the edge of the film where the cardboard cover was placed. Turn on all of the safelights normally used in the darkroom.

3.   Expose the first one-inch strip for one minute to the safelight illumination. Following the first exposure, slide the cardboard down approximately one additional inch, mark film edge and expose for another minute. Expose five successive one-inch sections at 1-minute intervals following the same procedure. Leave a one-inch strip on the bottom unexposed to any safelight. This procedure produces strips of the film with 0 through 7 minutes of safelight exposure.

4.   Turn off all safelights and process the film.

5.   Record densitometer readings on both halves of all the one-inch sections of the test film. When the film is processed, the exposed side should yield a density in the 0.35–1.0 density range. The film is **unacceptable** if the density is not within the above range and the procedure should be repeated with an appropriate adjustment of exposure factors.

RESULTS

Time Exposed to Safelight	Optical Density	
	Exposed Half	Unexposed Half
7 min	_____	_____
6 min	_____	_____
5 min	_____	_____
4 min	_____	_____
3 min	_____	_____
2 min	_____	_____
1 min	_____	_____
0 min	_____	_____

ANALYSIS

1. Describe the effects of safelight illumination on radiographic density. How close do the densitometric results agree with your visual observations?

2. Did the exposed and non-exposed sides of the film respond equally to the test? If different, how?

3. Based on your results, would you estimate that film in the film bin or an exposed film would be more sensitive to darkroom safelight fog? If different, what do you believe would cause the difference?

4. How could you determine whether the fog received was due to safelights or to light leaks around openings?

5. What is the safelight filter type used in the experiment? List the bulb wattage and approximate distance from the film for the safelight(s) used.

WORKSHEET 31–1   **COMPARING EXPOSURE SYSTEMS**

PURPOSE

Compare various types of exposure systems.

ACTIVITIES

Answer the following questions:

1. What is the goal of a radiographic exposure system?

2. How do radiographic exposure systems function (generically) to achieve this goal?

3. Describe a fixed optimum kilovoltage exposure system.

4. List at least three advantages and three disadvantages associated with this type of system.

5. Describe a variable kilovoltage exposure system.

6. List at least three advantages and three disadvantages associated with this type of system.

7. Describe an automatic exposure control (AEC) exposure system.

8. List at least three advantages and three disadvantages associated with this type of system.

9. List three other exposure systems and briefly describe what makes them distinctive.

10.   Fill in the missing steps in the establishment of a technique chart.

ESTABLISHING A TECHNIQUE CHART

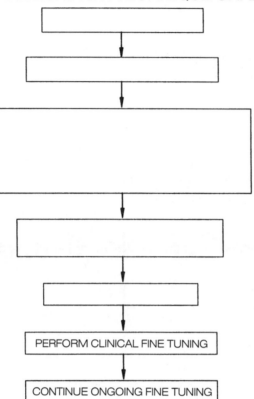

PERFORM CLINICAL FINE TUNING

CONTINUE ONGOING FINE TUNING

WORKSHEET 31–2   **ESTABLISHING A TECHNIQUE CHART**

PURPOSE

Establish a technique chart.

ACTIVITIES

Use the following scenarios to answer the questions below.

Scenario 1. A newly constructed orthopedic clinic has hired you to run a one radiology room. The radiographic unit is a 500 mA single-phase generator and is not equipped with automatic exposure control. A rare earth image receptor system is being used. One of your initial duties will be to establish a technique chart to be used in the facility. The manager of the clinic is willing to provide you with any of the resources that you will need to accomplish this task.

1.   What type of exposure system are you going to use in developing your technique chart? Justify your decision.

2.   You will begin the production of your technique chart by developing techniques for a lumbar spine. Describe the steps you would take to establish a reliable technique chart for lumbar spine examinations.

Scenario 2. You are responsible for a quality control program in a ten-room radiology department in a 400-bed community hospital. The department includes five general diagnostic rooms (including one dedicated chest unit and one room with tomography), three radiographic and fluoroscopic (R&F) rooms equipped with spot film and 105 mm photo-spot film devices, a special procedures room capable of bi-plane angiography, and one emergency radiology suite (located in the diagnostic area). All the generators are three phase or high frequency and equipped with automatic exposure controls, except the ER suite which is single phase without automatic exposure control. A 400 RS rare earth imaging system is currently being used. You have been charged with developing a technique system to be used in the facility. The department head is willing to provide you with any of the resources that you will need to accomplish this task.

3.   What type of exposure system will you use to develop your technique chart? Justify your decision.

4.   Describe the steps you would take to establish a reliable technique system for use in the general diagnostic area.

5.   After developing technique charts for the general diagnostic area, how would you go about designing a technique chart for use in the ER suite?

LABORATORY 32–1 _____ **DEVELOPING A FIXED kVp TECHNIQUE CHART**

PURPOSE

Construct a fixed kVp technique chart.

MATERIALS

1. Energized radiographic unit
2. Automatic film processor
3. Abdomen phantom
4. 14" x 17" radiographic cassettes with film

PROCEDURES

1. Position the abdomen phantom for an AP projection and measure its thickness at the CR entrance point.

2. Determine appropriate technical factors for a diagnostic quality image, expose, and process a film.

3. Evaluate the quality of the image. Repeat step 2 until a satisfactory diagnostic quality image is achieved. Record the exposure factors used on all radiographs along with the words "fixed kVp."

4. Produce four more images of the phantom using two different kVp levels above and two different kVp levels below the kVp used on the first image. Use the 15% rule or any other technique compensation system to adjust the mAs to compensate for the kVp changes. Repeat the films until all four radiographs display the same radiographic density as the first one.

5. Review all five of the test radiographs and eliminate the ones that you believe unacceptable. Of the radiographs remaining, the one with the highest kVp will be considered the optimal image. Write "optimal image" on this film. The kVp used to produce the "optimal image" is the fixed optimal kVp for that body part.

6. Complete the fixed kVp technique chart in the results section by extrapolating the required mAs values for the different part thickness based on the mAs used to obtain the optimal image.

RESULTS

FIXED kVp TECHNIQUE CHART

PART _____

PROJECTION _____

_____ kVp

_____ " SID

_____ Relative Speed

_____ Table Top

_____ Grid/Bucky

_____ Grid Ratio

COMMENTS:

cm	mAs
16	
17	
18	
19	
20	
21	
22	
23	
24	
25	
26	
27	
28	
29	
30	
31	
32	
33	

ANALYSIS

1. Based on your experience in this laboratory, discuss the fixed kVp approach to technique development with respect to accuracy, quality of results, ease of use, and usefulness in modifying established techniques.

2. Based on your experience, discuss the advantages and disadvantages of using the fixed kVp system in a clinical situation.

LABORATORY 33-1   **DEVELOPING A VARIABLE kVp TECHNIQUE CHART**

PURPOSE

Construct a variable kVp technique chart.

MATERIALS

1. Energized radiographic unit
2. Automatic film processor
3. Abdomen phantom
4. 14" x 17" radiographic cassettes with film

PROCEDURES

1. Position the abdomen phantom for an AP projection and measure its thickness at the CR entrance point.

2. Determine the kVp to be used according to the (cm x 2) + 30 kVp formula. Choose a mAs value, based on the body part, part thickness, kVp, and SID that you feel will produce a diagnostic quality image. Expose and process a film.

3. Evaluate the quality of the image. Repeat step 2 until a satisfactory diagnostic quality image is achieved. Record the exposure factors used on all radiographs and label them "standard variable kVp."

4. Produce four more images of the phantom using two different kVp levels above and two different kVp levels below the kVp used on the first image. Use the 15% rule or any other technique compensation system to adjust the mAs to compensate for the kVp changes. Repeat the films until all four radiographs display the same radiographic density as the first one.

5. Review all five of the test radiographs and eliminate the ones that you believe unacceptable (pay particular attention to the contrast). Of the radiographs remaining, the one with the highest kVp will be considered the low contrast limit and the one with the lowest kVp will be considered the high contrast limit. All the radiographs between these limits would presumably have acceptable contrast, assuming the radiographic density is adequate. Record the kVp values that represent the chosen limits.

6. Complete the variable kVp technique chart in the results section, by extrapolating the required kVp values for the different part thickness based on a 2 kVp change per cm thickness. During the extrapolation when the kVp reaches either the low or high contrast limit recorded earlier, adjust the kVp (with the appropriate mAs compensation) to bring it back to the beginning of the acceptable contrast range, then continue the extrapolation.

RESULTS

VARIABLE kVp TECHNIQUE CHART

PART _____

PROJECTION _____

_____ " SID

_____ Relative Speed

_____ Table Top

_____ Grid/Bucky

_____ Grid Ratio

COMMENTS:

cm	kVp	mAs
16		
17		
18		
19		
20		
21		
22		
23		
24		
25		
26		
27		
28		
29		
30		
31		
32		
33		

ANALYSIS

1. Based on your experience in this laboratory, discuss the variable kVp approach to technique development with respect to accuracy, quality of results, ease of use, and usefulness in modifying established techniques.

2. Based on your experience, discuss the advantages and disadvantages of using the variable kVp system in a clinical situation.

WORKSHEET 34-1 _____ **USING THE DU PONT BIT SYSTEM**

PURPOSE

Use the bit system to convert exposure factors.

ACTIVITIES

Use the Du Pont Bit System for the following questions (see appendix C of the textbook or request a current copy of the Bit System chart from a Du Pont representative).

The following technical exposure factors produce a high quality diagnostic radiograph of a healthy adult male patient. Use this technique as the basis for answering all the questions.

<u>AP ABDOMEN</u>

	Bits				Bits	
kVp:	70	= _____	Collimation:	14" x 17"	= _____
mAs:	80	= _____	Relative Speed:	200	= _____
FFD:	40"	= _____	Patient Size:	20 cm	= _____
Grid:	8:1 80 LPI	= _____	Generator:	1 Phase	= _____
Bucky Space:	2"	= _____		TOTAL BITS	_____

1. Calculate the Bit value for each of the exposure variables along with the total number of Bits and fill in the blanks above with your answers.

2. What new mAs would be necessary to compensate for lower contrast if the kVp was increased to 85?

3. What new mAs would be necessary to compensate for a change to an 800 RS film/screen system?

4. What mAs would be necessary for a patient measuring 23 cm?

5. What kVp would be necessary to compensate for using a three-phase, 12 pulse generator while maintaining the contrast?

6. What mAs would be necessary to compensate for changing to a 12:1, 103 LPI grid?

7. What kVp adjustment would be necessary to compensate for a patient with ascites?

8. What mAs would be necessary to compensate for changing to an AP spot film of L2–L3 with an extension cone?

LABORATORY 34-2

USING THE SIEMENS POINT SYSTEM

PURPOSE

Utilize the Siemens Point System to develop a fixed kilovoltage technique chart.

MATERIALS

1. Energized radiographic unit
2. Automatic film processor
3. Phantom body parts
4. Radiographic cassettes with film (various sizes)

PROCEDURES

1. Select an appropriate phantom and set the suggested technical exposure factors from the Siemens Point System for one projection (see appendix D of the textbook or request a current copy of the Siemens Point System chart from a Siemens representative). Read across the table to the points column. This point total is the logarithmic sum of the various exposure factor variables used, i.e., SID, grid ratio, etc.

2. Make the necessary point adjustments to make the exposure table applicable for the equipment being used. Refer to the Correction Values table and either add or subtract the appropriate exposure points to the total as necessary (i.e., adjust for differences in relative speed, grid ratio, generator, etc.). For this activity, consider 40" to be equivalent to 105 cm. A Siemens Pb 12/40 grid can be described as 12:1 ratio/40 lines per cm. Record all adjustments in the results section.

3. Measure the thickness of the phantom at the CR entrance point. Consider the phantom to be a normal average adult. If the phantom thickness differs from the thickness given in the exposure table for the projection, adjust 1 point per cm difference.

4. After all point adjustments have been made, use the new point total to determine the kVp and mAs for the projection. Refer to the Correction Table to convert exposure points into kVp and mAs. Take the exam points total and distribute it appropriately between kVp and mAs points [i.e., if the exam total is 30 points, then 70 kVp (13 points) and 50 mAs (17 points) would be appropriate as would be 81 kVp (16 points) and 25 mAs (24 points)].

5. Position the phantom, expose and process the film. Record the technical exposure factors on the radiograph along with the words "fixed kVp."

6. Evaluate the density of the radiograph. Repeat the film with appropriate mAs adjustments until a satisfactory image is obtained. Label the film "standard."

7. Record the final exposure factors for the standard radiograph and add techniques for patient sizes on either side of the average.

RESULTS

FIXED kVp TECHNIQUE CHART

PART _____

PROJECTION _____

_____ kVp

_____ " SID

_____ Relative Speed

_____ Table Top

_____ Grid/Bucky

_____ Grid Ratio

COMMENTS:

cm Thickness	mAs

ANALYSIS

1. Discuss the Siemens Point System approach to technique development with respect to accuracy, quality of results, ease of use, and use in modifying established techniques.

2. Discuss the advantages and disadvantages of using the Siemens Point System in a clinical situation.

LABORATORY 34–3   USING PROPORTIONAL ANATOMY CONSTANTS

PURPOSE

Develop a technique chart using proportional anatomy constants.

MATERIALS

1. Energized radiographic unit
2. Automatic film processor
3. Abdomen and skull phantom
4. 14" x 17" and 10" x 12" radiographic cassettes with film

PROCEDURES

1. Measure an abdomen phantom just below the tip of the sternum. Refer to the Kilovoltage vs. Measured Centimeter Thickness Chart (Table 33–4) in the textbook and locate the measured part thickness in the center (cm) column. Read across the row to find the recommended kVp by using the scale column that is appropriate for the generator being used (scale 1 for three phase or high frequency, 1/2 scale for single phase).

2. Position the phantom for an AP lumbar spine projection. Using the recommended kVp, select a mAs value that will produce an acceptable density (OD 1.2 ± 0.1 in the psoas muscle area), expose, and process the film.

3. Review the radiograph and evaluate its density. Adjust the mAs appropriately and repeat until a diagnostic image is produced. Record the exposure factors and label the film "standard." The mAs becomes a constant mAs ratio for further calculations.

4. Refer to the mAs Ratio Chart (Table 33–5) in the textbook and find the mAs ratio for a lateral skull. Calculate the mAs required for the lateral skull by substituting the lateral skull mAs ratio and the mAs used for the AP lumber spine (step 4) in the mAs ratio formula:

$$\frac{\text{mAs for body part}}{\text{mAs for AP lumbar}} = \text{mAs ratio for body part}$$

5. Select the recommended kVp for the lateral skull: (1) refer to the mAs Ratio Chart (Table 33–5 in textbook) to find the appropriate scale for the generator, (2) measure the phantom skull for a lateral projection, (3) refer to the Kilovoltage vs. Measured Centimeter Thickness Chart (Table 33–4) and use the measured thickness and the appropriate scale to locate the recommended kVp.

6. Position the phantom skull for a lateral projection, use the recommended mAs and kVp, expose, and process the film.

7. Review the radiograph, adjust the mAs appropriately, and repeat if necessary until an optimal diagnostic image is produced. Record the exposure factors and label the film "standard."

8. Extrapolate the required kVp values for the different part thicknesses based on the Kilovoltage vs. Measured Centimeter Thickness Chart (Table 33–4) and complete the variable kVp technique chart in the results section.

RESULTS

1. AP Lumbar Spine _____ cm _____Scale _____ kVp _____mAs

2. AP LAT Skull _____ mAs ratio _____mAs _____Scale _____cm _____kVp

VARIABLE kVp TECHNIQUE CHART

PART _____

PROJECTION _____

_____ " SID

_____ Relative Speed

_____ Table Top

_____ Grid/Bucky

_____ Grid Ratio

COMMENTS:

cm	kVp	mAs
12		
13		
14		
15		
16		
17		
18		
19		
20		

ANALYSIS

1. How effective is the proportional anatomy constant system?

2. How could you utilize this system in establishing a clinical technique chart?

3. Compare this approach to technique conversion according to the fixed kVp system; the variable kVp system; the Du Pont Bit System; the Siemens Point System.

LABORATORY 35–1   DETERMINING AND CONTROLLING ION CHAMBER CONFIGURATIONS

PURPOSE

Demonstrate the configuration and correct selection of ion chambers in an automatic exposure control device.

MATERIALS

1. Energized radiographic unit equipped with ion chamber automatic exposure control
2. Automatic film processor
3. 14" x 17" cassette with film matched to AEC system being tested
4. Abdomen or pelvis phantom

SUGGESTED EXPOSURE FACTORS

400 RS, 100 mA, phototimed, 80 kVp, 40" SID, 8:1 Bucky grid

PROCEDURES

1. Set the tube to 40" SID, center to the table, place a loaded 14" x 17" cassette in the Bucky tray, align to the central ray, and collimate beam to the film size.

2. Set the generator for manual technique control [deactivate the automatic exposure device (phototimer)], expose, and process the film.

3. Evaluate the image carefully to see if the location of the ion chambers can be visualized (faintly). Repeat the film with appropriate mAs adjustments if necessary.

4. Set the tube to 40" SID, center to the table, position the phantom for an AP projection, place a loaded 14" x 17" cassette in the Bucky tray, align to the central ray, and collimate to the film size.

5. Select the normal density setting for the AEC system, use an mA station that is normally used with the AEC (usually 100 to 400 mA), use 80 kVp, select the center sensing chamber, expose, and process the film.

6. Produce another film by repeating steps 4 and 5 with one of the lateral sensing chambers selected.

7. Produce another film by repeating steps 4 and 5 with all three sensing chambers selected.

RESULTS

1. Review the first film and draw an arrow to the edges of each ion chamber.

2. Review the other images with respect to their radiographic density and contrast.

ANALYSIS

1. How many ion chambers were demonstrated on the first film? Are all the chambers of the same size?

2. Does the configuration of the chambers match the configuration demonstrated on the collimator template? If not or if there is no indication of chamber location on the collimator, describe the configuration in terms relevant to their use while positioning patients.

3. Describe the density and contrast differences of the last three films.

4. Which radiograph would be the most appropriate for an abdominal survey procedure? Why?

5. Which would be the most appropriate for a lumbar spine procedure? Why?

LABORATORY 35-2   THE EFFECT OF POSITIONING ON AUTOMATIC EXPOSURE CONTROL

PURPOSE

Demonstrate the effect of positioning errors on the image quality of automatic exposure control radiographs.

MATERIALS

1. Energized radiographic unit with automatic exposure control
2. Automatic film processor
3. 14" x 17" cassette with film matched to AEC system being tested
4. Abdomen or pelvis phantom

SUGGESTED EXPOSURE FACTORS

400 RS, 400 mA, phototimed, 80 kVp, 40" SID, 8:1 Bucky grid

PROCEDURES

1. Set the tube to a 40" SID, center to the table, position the phantom for a lateral lumbar spine, place a loaded 14" x 17" cassette in the Bucky tray, align to the central ray, and collimate to the spine (approximately 6" x 17").

2. Select the normal density setting for the AEC system, use an mA station that is normally used with the AEC (usually 100 to 400 mA), use 80 kVp, select the center chamber, expose, and process the film.

3. Produce a second radiograph by repeating steps 1 and 2 with the phantom moved 1.5" posteriorly.

4. Produce a third radiograph by repeating steps 1 and 2 with the phantom moved 1.5" anteriorly.

RESULTS

1. Review the three radiographs with respect to radiographic density and contrast.

ANALYSIS

1. Which film exhibits the best image quality? Why?

2. Which film exhibits the worst image quality? Why?

3.   What caused the image quality to change between the first and second films?

4.   What caused the image quality to change between the first and third films?

LABORATORY 35–3   THE EFFECT OF COLLIMATION ON AUTOMATIC EXPOSURE CONTROL

PURPOSE

Demonstrate the effects and control of scatter radiation on automatic exposure control radiographs.

MATERIALS

1. Energized radiographic unit equipped with automatic exposure control
2. Automatic film processor
3. 14" x 17" cassette with film matched to AEC system being tested
4. Abdomen or pelvis phantom
5. Lead masks

SUGGESTED EXPOSURE FACTORS

400 RS, 400 mA, phototimed, 80 kVp, 40" SID, 8:1 Bucky grid

PROCEDURES

1. Set the tube to a 40" SID, center to the table, position the phantom for a lateral lumbar spine, place a loaded 14" x 17" cassette in the Bucky tray, align to the central ray, and collimate to the film size.

2. Select the normal density setting for the AEC system, use an mA station that is normally used with the AEC (usually 100 to 400 mA), use 80 kVp, select the center ion chamber, expose, and process the film.

3. Produce a second radiograph by repeating steps 1 and 2 with the beam collimated to the lumbar spine (6" x 17").

4. Produce a third radiograph by repeating steps 1 and 2 with the beam collimated to the lumbar spine (6" x 17") with the addition of lead masks on the table to outline the posterior aspect of the soft tissue. Position the lead masks carefully so as not to overlap the posterior aspect of the phantom.

RESULTS

1. Review the three radiographs with respect to radiographic density and contrast.

ANALYSIS

1. Which film exhibits the best image quality? Why?

2.   Which film exhibits the worst image quality? Why?

3.   What caused the image quality to change between the first and second films?

4.   What caused the image quality to change between the second and third films?

LABORATORY 35-4   **EVALUATING AUTOMATIC EXPOSURE CONTROLS**

PURPOSE

Evaluate the performance of automatic exposure control kVp compensation and response capability.

MATERIALS

1.   Energized radiographic unit with automatic exposure control
2.   Automatic film processor
3.   Two aluminum (1100 alloy) plates 7" x 7" x 3/4"
4.   One cassette with film matched to AEC system being tested
5.   Densitometer
6.   Lead identification markers

SUGGESTED EXPOSURE FACTORS

See Procedure.

PROCEDURES

1.   Set the tube to a 40" SID, center to the table, position one Al plate to the center of the light field, and collimate the field to slightly less than the dimensions of the aluminum plate. Place the lead markers along the edge of the field to label the film #1.

2.   Place a loaded cassette in the Bucky tray, align to the central ray, select the normal density setting for the AEC system, use an mA station that is normally used with the AEC (usually 100 to 400 mA), use 70 kVp, select the center chamber, expose, and process the film.

3.   Using the same cassette, repeat steps 1 and 2, label the film #2, but use 85 kVp. Repeat the procedure again labeling the film #3 and using 100 kVp.

4.   Place the second Al plate on top of the first and repeat procedures 1 through 3, labeling the films #3, 4, and 5.

RESULTS

1.   Measure the optical densities of the six films in the center of each image with a densitometer and record the readings below as a function of kVp vs. thickness of aluminum.

	0.75" Al	1.5" Al
70 kVp	_____	_____
85 kVp	_____	_____
100 kVp	_____	_____

2. Evaluate the test data against an acceptance criteria of ± OD 0.20 for the kVp compensation and response capability tests.

ANALYSIS

1. Do your test results meet the acceptance criteria for the parameters tested?

2. What might be some possible problems with the AEC device that would cause the densities to exceed the acceptance criteria for these tests?

3. What is meant by the minimum response time of an AEC system?

4. What is the purpose of the backup timer in an AEC system?

5. It has been suggested that a fixed kVp exposure technique system be used with AEC devices when using rare earth imaging systems. Defend this statement.

WORKSHEET 36-1   **SOLVING MULTIPLE EFFECTS PROBLEMS**

PURPOSE

Practice solving multiple effect exposure problems.

ACTIVITIES

Select the set of exposure factors that would produce the greatest radiographic density for questions 1–7.

		mA	mAs	Time	kVp	SID	Screens (Relative Speed)	Grid
1.	(a)	100	20	1/5 sec	65			
	(b)	200	20	1/10 sec	70			
	(c)	50	20	2/5 sec	65			
	(d)	400	20	1/20 sec	60			
2.	(a)	300	12	0.04 sec		40"		
	(b)	600	15	0.025 sec		36"		
	(c)	800	12	0.015 sec		40"		
	(d)	200	10	0.05 sec		36"		
3.	(a)	100	10	1/10 sec	68	36"		
	(b)	75	15	1/5 sec	68	36"		
	(c)	400	10	1/20 sec	68	36"		
	(d)	600	5	1/60 sec	68	36"		
4.	(a)	500	5	0.02 sec	80		100	
	(b)	1000	4	0.01 sec	75		100	
	(c)	300	5	0.05 sec	80		100	
	(d)	600	40	0.033 sec	75		100	
5.	(a)	500	100	1/5 sec				8:1
	(b)	1000	100	1/10 sec				12:1
	(c)	1000	125	1/8 sec				8:1
	(d)	500	125	1/4 sec				12:1
6.	(a)	400	60	150 msec	75	36"	200	12:1
	(b)	500	26	80 msec	75	36"	200	16:1
	(c)	800	30	150 msec	75	36"	200	12:1
	(d)	1500	60	20 msec	75	36"	200	8:1
7.	(a)	200	132	1/20 sec	65	40"	100	8:1
	(b)	150	15	1/10 sec	60	50"	100	8:1
	(c)	300	132	1/30 sec	65	50"	100	8:1
	(d)	200	20	1/10 sec	60	60"	100	8:1

8. A satisfactory radiograph is produced using a single-phase, fully rectified generator, 75 kVp, 200 mA, 0.10 sec, 40" SID, 400 RS, and an 8:1 grid. What exposure time would be required to produce a new radiograph with the same density if a three-phase, twelve-pulse generator, 100 mA, 100 RS, and 5:1 grid are used?

9. A satisfactory radiograph is produced using a three-phase, twelve-pulse generator, 60 kVp, 6.6 mAs, 36" SID, 100 RS, without a grid. What mAs would be required to produce a new radiograph with the same density if a three-phase, six-pulse generator, 65 kVp, 40" SID, 400 RS, and an 8:1 grid are used?

10. A satisfactory radiograph is produced for a 20 cm AP pelvis using a three-phase, twelve-pulse generator, 80 kVp, 30 mAs, 40" SID, 300 RS, and a 12:1 grid. What mAs would be required to produce a new radiograph with the same density for a 24 cm AP pelvis if a single-phase, two-pulse generator, 92 kVp, 60" SID, 800 RS, and 5:1 grid are used?

LABORATORY 37-1   THE EFFECT OF ALIGNMENT AND DISTANCE
                                       ON MOBILE RADIOGRAPHIC IMAGE QUALITY

PURPOSE

Demonstrate the effect of central ray alignment and distance on image quality during mobile procedures.

MATERIALS

1. Energized radiographic unit
2. Automatic film processor
3. 10" x 12" cassette with film
4. Coconut (milk-filled) (when buying coconut, shake to hear milk)

SUGGESTED EXPOSURE FACTORS

400 RS, 100 mA, 0.05 sec, 5 mAs, 50 kVp, 40" SID

PROCEDURES

ALIGNMENT PROBLEMS

1. Place the coconut in the center of a 10" x 12" cassette, direct the central ray to the center of the cassette, collimate to the film size, set the tube to a 40" SID, label the film #1, expose, and process the film.

2. Place the cassette in a vertical position, label the film #2, and use a horizontal beam to repeat step 1 (use sponges as necessary to place the coconut in the center of the film).

3. Place the cassette on a 45 degree angle to the plane of the floor, label the film #3, and use a horizontal beam to repeat step 1.

4. Place the cassette on a 45 degree angle to the plane of the floor, label the film #4, direct the central ray perpendicular to the film, and repeat step 1.

ESTIMATING DISTANCE

1. Conceal the distance indicator on the radiographic unit, estimate a 36" SID, then reveal the distance indicator and record the actual SID.

2. Repeat step 1 estimating 40", 56", and 72" SIDs.

DISTANCE/DENSITY PROBLEMS

1. Place the coconut in the center of a 10" x 12" cassette, direct the central ray to the center of the cassette, collimate to the film size, set the tube to a 36" SID, label the film #5, expose, and process the film.

2. Repeat step 1, using a 38" SID for film #6, a 40" SID for film #7, and a 42" SID for film #8.

RESULTS

ESTIMATING DISTANCE

1. Record the actual distance for the following estimated distances:

    36" SID   _____
    40" SID   _____
    56" SID   _____
    72" SID   _____

ANALYSIS

ALIGNMENT PROBLEMS

1. Review films #1–4. Which of the images demonstrate a sharp air-fluid level within the coconut?

2. What is the proper procedure to demonstrate air-fluid levels in a patient?

3. What effects do film and tube placement have on the demonstration of air-fluid levels?

ESTIMATING DISTANCE

4. How close were the actual distances to the estimated distances?

5. What effect will estimating distance for a mobile procedure have on image quality?

DISTANCE/DENSITY PROBLEMS

6. Review films #5–8. What effects do small changes in distance have on radiographic density?

7. How much of a distance change is necessary to notice the effect of the change on the image?

LABORATORY 38–1 OPERATING FLUOROSCOPIC SPOT FILMING SYSTEMS

PURPOSE

Operate a fluoroscopic spot filming system.

MATERIALS

1. Energized fluoroscopic unit
2. Lead apron
3. Spot film camera or spot film cassettes
4. Large radiographic phantom (i.e., chest, abdomen, or pelvis)
5. Automatic film processor

EXPOSURE FACTORS

Suggested Factors

Medium mA (by setting brightness control) at 70–120 kVp

PROCEDURES

1. Wearing a lead apron, place the phantom at the center of the fluoroscopic unit and move the carriage into the operating position.

2. Use the foot pedal to turn the fluoroscope on. Move the carriage until the phantom is centered to the image.

3. Use the carriage controls to set the spot film system to a 4 on 1 position and make two spot film exposures. Move the carriage slightly and then set the spot film system to a 2 on 1 position so that a single exposure will completely fill the remaining portion of the film. Make the exposure and process the film.

RESULTS

1. Mark the film to show which exposure was made first, second, and third.

ANALYSIS

1. Draw each of the possible spot film exposure configurations available on the fluoroscopic unit that was used.

2. Describe at least one clinical examination for which each of the following spot film configurations would be most useful: 4 on 1, 2 on 1 vertical, 2 on 1 horizontal, and 1 on 1.

LABORATORY 38-2   FLUOROSCOPIC AUTOMATIC BRIGHTNESS CONTROLS

PURPOSE

Explain the basic function of a fluoroscopic automatic brightness control.

MATERIALS

1. Energized fluoroscopic unit
2. Lead apron
3. Spot film camera or spot film cassettes
4. Large radiographic phantom (i.e., chest, abdomen, or pelvis)
5. Automatic film processor

EXPOSURE FACTORS

Suggested Factors

Medium mA (by setting brightness control) at 70–120 kVp

PROCEDURES

1. Wearing a lead apron, place the phantom at the center of the fluoroscopic unit and move the carriage into the operating position.

2. Use the foot pedal to turn the fluoroscope on. Move the carriage until the phantom is centered to the image.

3. Move the carriage slowly from the center of the phantom to one side, observing the image closely during the motion.

4. Return the carriage slowly to the center of the phantom and then move it gradually up or down until the phantom disappears from the image.

ANALYSIS

1. Describe how the image changes as the fluoroscope moves from a thick portion of the phantom to a thin region.

2.   Explain the mechanism that causes the changes described in #1.

LABORATORY 39-1

TOMOGRAPHIC DEPTH AND THICKNESS

PURPOSE

Determine the location and thickness of a tomographic focal plane.

MATERIALS

1. Energized tomographic unit
2. Automatic film processor
3. 8" x 10" cassette with film
4. Tomographic phantom (commercial or homemade). Typically consists of a number of acrylic discs. One disc contains lead numbers spaced 1 mm apart arranged in a helix so as to indicate slice level and thickness. One disc contains different size mesh pieces to evaluate focal plane resolution. Several discs of different thicknesses to be used as spacers. Lead disc with a 4 mm aperture in the center to evaluate beam uniformity and path.

SUGGESTED EXPOSURE FACTORS

200 RS, 60 mAs, 70 kVp, 40" SID, 8:1 Bucky grid

PROCEDURES

1. Center the 4 cm spacer on the table. Place the number helix disc on top of it followed by the 1 and 2 cm spacer discs.

2. Adjust the fulcrum of the system for 4.5 cm (45 mm).

3. Place 8" x 10" cassette in Bucky tray and collimate beam to film size.

4. Set the tomographic angle (arc) to the maximum routinely used. Make sure the exposure time is long enough to cover the complete tomographic arc.

5. Expose and process the film.

RESULTS

1. Review the test radiograph in terms of image blur of the lead numbers.

2. Identify the lead number that demonstrates the least blur (in best focus). This represents the level of the fulcrum and the focal plane.

3. The focal plane (section level) should be within ± 2.5 mm of the fulcrum for linear motion and ± 1 mm for pluridirectional motion.

4. Identify the range of lead numbers that demonstrate partial blurring (in focus). This represents the section thickness (focal plane thickness). Numbers that appear completely blurred are outside of the focal plane.

5. The section thickness varies with tomographic angle, but a linear sweep with a 30 degree arc should have a section thickness of 2 to 2.5 mm. A multi-directional unit operating in excess of 30 degrees should have a section thickness of about 1 mm. Consult the unit operating manual for a table of section thicknesses.

ANALYSIS

1. Which lead number demonstrates the least blur? Does this represent the level of the fulcrum? Explain.

2. What is the range of numbers that you consider to be in focus (slightly or partially blurred)? What is the section thickness demonstrated?

3. Does this seem reasonable based on the tomographic angle used? Explain.

4. Explain why the level of the fulcrum should demonstrate the plane with the least amount of blur (best focus).

5. Explain why the tomographic angle determines the thickness of the section (focal plane).

3f

LABORATORY 39-2   TOMOGRAPHIC MOTION

PURPOSE

Determine the path of the x-ray beam during a tomographic exposure.

MATERIALS

1. Energized tomographic unit
2. Automatic film processor
3. 8" x 10" cassette with film
4. Tomographic phantom (commercial or homemade). Typically consists of a number of acrylic discs. One disc contains lead numbers spaced 1 mm apart arranged in a helix so as to indicate slice level and thickness. One disc contains different size mesh pieces to evaluate focal plane resolution. Several discs of different thicknesses to be used as spacers. Lead disc with a 4 mm aperture in the center to evaluate beam uniformity and path.

SUGGESTED EXPOSURE FACTORS

200 RS, 60 mAs, 70 kVp, 40" SID, 8:1 Bucky grid

PROCEDURES

1. Center the 4 cm spacer disc on the table, followed by the 1 and 2 cm spacers. Center the lead aperture disc on top of the stack of spacers.

2. Adjust the fulcrum of the system for 4.5 cm (45 mm).

3. Place 8" x 10" cassette in Bucky tray and collimate beam to film size.

4. With the x-ray tube centered and perpendicular to the film, make a non-tomographic exposure at the same kVp and about 10% of the mAs needed to properly expose the phantom. This exposure will mark the center of the pinhole trace.

5. Set the angle (arc) to the maximum routinely used. Make sure the exposure time is long enough to cover the complete tomographic arc and produce a tomographic exposure of the phantom.

6. Repeat the procedure in the opposite direction for linear tomographic equipment that exposes in both directions.

7. Process and evaluate the film. Depending on the phantom thickness, the pinhole trace may be too dark to interpret. An ideal density would be approximately 1.0, although it can vary greatly. A better exposure can be achieved by varying the number of spacers used. Repeat steps 1–7 if necessary to obtain an image.

RESULTS

1. Review the test radiograph image for completeness and uniformity.

2. The image pattern represents the path of the beam during exposure.

3. The beam path should follow a smooth, uniform course. For linear tomography the beam path image should be equally divided on either side of the center (exposure) mark. Multidirectional units should not produce gaps or overlaps on the beam path image greater than 10% of the beam path length.

4. The optical density of the beam path image represents the uniformity of the exposure.

5. The density of the beam path should demonstrate minimal variations (less than 0.3 OD). Areas of increased and decreased density may indicate hesitation or changes in the speed of the tomographic sweep.

ANALYSIS

1. Does the image pattern of the tomographic phantom represent the tomographic motion used? Describe and explain.

2. Does the beam path image meet the criteria for completeness of motion? Describe and explain.

3. Does the uniformity of exposure appear to be acceptable? Describe and explain.

4. Explain the clinical importance of completeness and uniformity of tube motion during a tomographic study.

PURPOSE

Explain differences between diagnostic radiography equipment and that specialized for mammography.

ACTIVITIES

1.   What are the primary reasons for considering high frequency generators for mammography?

2.   What is the kVp range utilized in mammography?

3.   Mammographic contrast must be sufficient to demonstrate microcalcifications that are extremely small. What is the size range that must be visualized adequately?

4.   What is the major disadvantage of using kVp in the 20s range?

5.   What is the typical mammography mA range?

6. What material is used for the target of mammography x-ray tube anodes?

7. What is the minimum HVL required by the U.S. government for 30 kVp?

8. What is the range of mammography grid ratios and frequencies?

WORKSHEET 41–1   **VASCULAR IMAGING EQUIPMENT**

PURPOSE

Explain differences between diagnostic radiography equipment and that specialized for vascular procedures.

ACTIVITIES

1.   What is the desirable mA range for a vascular x-ray generator?

2.   What is the desirable kVp range for a vascular x-ray generator?

3.   What is an appropriate continuous heat loading capability for an angiographic generator?

4.   What is indicated by a percent duty cycle chart?

5.   What is an appropriate time in motion value?

6.   What are the five factors that affect injector flow rate?

7. What is an ECG trigger?

WORKSHEET 42-1   **DIGITAL IMAGE PROCESSING**

PURPOSE

Describe the process of digital image data acquisition and reconstruction.

ACTIVITIES

1. If density measurements of the pixels in Figure A were made, they might be expressed as the numbers shown in Figure B. This is essentially a digitization of the information shown in Figure A.

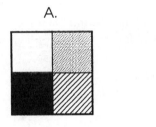

2. If the box is irradiated, the attenuation data received for various projections by adding the density values for each line of values within the pixels would appear as follows:

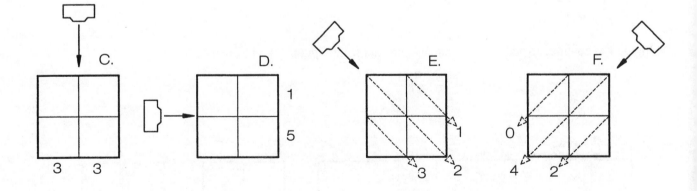

3. A computed tomography unit accumulates information in a much more complex, but similar, process. When considering only a single projection, the computer assumes that the density values for each pixel are equal as shown in Figure G.

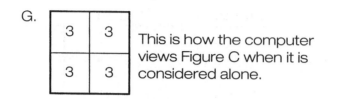

G.

This is how the computer views Figure C when it is considered alone.

Because this is obviously not accurate, it is necessary to develop a method for the computer to compare and weigh the information from each projection to obtain an accurate image.

4. To reconstruct the information in Figure B, which would then permit the image in Figure A to be created, the computer must backproject the attenuation data received for the various projections (Figures C, D, E, and F).

Using only the information given in Figures C, D, E, and F, total the attenuation for each pixel by summing the accumulated total for each projection as shown in Figure H.

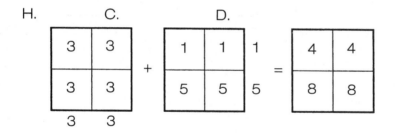

Use Figure I to continue to add the pixel attenuation data from Figures E and F.

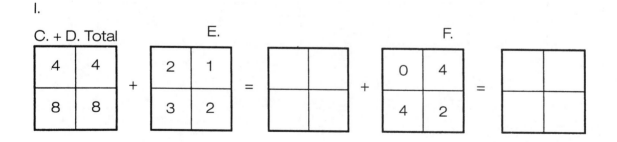

5. The information in Figure I can then be manipulated mathematically to reconstruct Figure B. First subtract the background value (the minimum number for any pixel), which is 6.

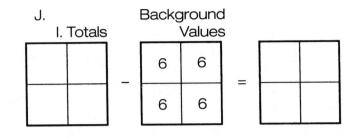

Then divide each pixel by 3 to reconstruct Figure B. This number is achieved in computed tomography by complex formulas based on many variables within the system.

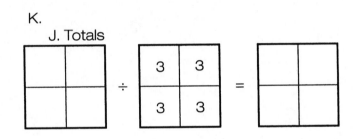

LABORATORY 42-2   **CONTROLLING AND EVALUATING DIGITAL IMAGES**

PURPOSE

Explain the function of digital image window level and width controls.

MATERIALS

1. Computed tomography or magnetic resonance imaging console

PROCEDURE

1. Request a technologist who is familiar with the operating console to bring up an average image and adjust it to diagnostic window levels. Have the technologist indicate which controls operate the image window level and width. Also have this technologist indicate which numbers on the CRT indicate the window level and width. Record these numbers for use during this laboratory.

2. Use only the window level control to make the image completely light. Record this number. Carefully observe the effect on the demonstration of various structures as the window level is slowly increased to complete darkness. Record this number. Bring the window level back to the original number. Watch the CRT closely while the window level is very slowly increased. Record the number when the first visible change is observed.

3. Use only the window width control to make the image completely light. Record this number. Carefully observe the effect on the demonstration of various structures as the window width is slowly increased to complete darkness. Record this number. Bring the window width back to the original number. Watch the CRT closely while the window width is very slowly increased. Record the number when the first visible change is observed.

RESULTS

1. Record the window level and width numbers as indicated in the procedures above.

2. Subtract the window level number for the light image from the dark image and record the result as the range (R). Subtract the window level number for the light image from the original diagnostic quality image and record the result as the diagnostic level (D). Use the formula D/R*100 to determine the percentage of window level that produced the diagnostic image.

3. Repeat this process for the window width numbers.

ANALYSIS

1. What visible image quality factor is changing as the window level is varied?

2. What visible image quality factor is changing as the window width is varied?

3. Which primary mathematical functions is the computer applying to the image pixel data as the window level is changed?

4. Which primary mathematical functions is the computer applying to the image pixel data as the window width is changed?

5. What percentage change was required to see a density change?

6. What percentage change was required to see a contrast change?

7. What percent of the total available range of density produced the diagnostic quality image?

8. What percent of the total available range of contrast produced the diagnostic quality image?

LABORATORY 43-1   EVALUATING COMPUTED TOMOGRAPHIC IMAGES

PURPOSE

Evaluate basic parameters of a computed tomography image.

MATERIALS

1. Images from a complete abdominal computed tomography examination with essentially normal anatomy
2. Magnifying glass

ANALYSIS

1. Use the magnifying glass to locate a single pixel within the image.

2. Use the scanogram to locate a transverse section that demonstrates both kidneys.

3. List the following structures on this transverse section from anterior to posterior:

    (a) vertebral body
    (b) liver
    (c) kidney (right and left)
    (d) aorta
    (e) vena cava

4. List the same structures from left to right.

LABORATORY 44–1   SAFETY PRECAUTIONS FOR MAGNETIC RESONANCE IMAGING SYSTEMS

PURPOSE

Discuss safety measures for protection of all persons who approach the MRI unit magnetic field.

MATERIALS

1. Magnetic resonance imaging unit
2. CRT monitor
3. Metal dog leash with strong loop hand hold
4. Set of keys

NOTE: Most MRI units have a CRT monitor somewhere near the control console. If a slightly moveable CRT is not available near the console, any portable CRT is acceptable (i.e., an oscilloscope or black and white TV).

PROCEDURES

1. Remove all watches, credit cards, and other ferromagnetic objects prior to entering the MRI scanning room. Leave only a set of keys in a pocket.

2. Obtain an image on a CRT immediately outside the scanning room (within the 5–20 Gauss range). Rotate the CRT and observe the effect of the MRI unit's magnetic field on the image.

    NOTE: Some strongly shielded units may require that the CRT be brought inside the scanning room. However, this should never be done without the direct supervision of an MRI technologist.

3. Enter the MRI scanning room with an MRI technologist. Without removing the keys from a pocket, move within 2 feet of the entrance to the bore of the magnet.

4. Take a strong grip on the metal dog chain hand hold and very slowly allow the metallic end of the chain to approach the entrance to the bore of the magnet. Remove the chain at least 10 feet from the magnet before carefully handing it to another person.

RESULTS

1. Describe the effect of the MRI unit's magnetic field on a CRT monitor, the keys in a pocket, and the metallic dog chain.

ANALYSIS

1. Explain the effect of the strong magnetic field from the MRI unit on the CRT monitor. Consider both the laws of magnetism and the function of the components of a CRT.

2.   Explain the effect of the MRI unit's magnetic field on the keys and dog chain.

3.   By what factor does the magnetic force field increase as objects approach the bore of the magnet?

LABORATORY 44–2   EVALUATING MAGNETIC RESONANCE IMAGES

PURPOSE

Evaluate basic parameters of a magnetic resonance image.

MATERIALS

1. Images from a complete abdominal magnetic resonance imaging examination with essentially normal anatomy imaged in transverse, sagittal, and coronal images

2. Images from a complete abdominal computed tomography examination with essentially normal anatomy (MRI and CT images may be from different patients)

ANALYSIS

1. Locate the following structures on transverse, sagittal, and coronal sections:

    (a) vertebral body
    (b) liver
    (c) kidney
    (d) aorta
    (e) vena cava

2. Name an area that appears dark as a result of a signal void.

3. Describe the differences in the image of a vertebral body on the MR image with the CT image.

4. Describe the differences in the image of muscles on the MR image with the CT image.

225